No-Nonsense Oral Surgery

The ultimate guide to achieving oral surgery mastery for general dentists

Abdul Dalghous PhD (Leeds); BDS; MDentSci; FFD RCSI (OSOM); FDS RCS (Edinburgh); FDS RCPS (Glasgow); FDS RCS (England).

Specialist in Oral Surgery.
Founder and CEO of Yorkshire Dental Suite Leeds, UK.

Contents

This book is dedicated to my late father-in-law
Mr Aref Elhamedi.

Preface

This book of oral surgery is aimed at general and newly qualified dentists who are interested in teeth extraction. It is not for dental students or graduates preparing for membership or a speciality exam.

It does not cover everything in oral surgery, and is by no means a replacement of academic textbooks.

It summarises my vast experience in oral and maxillofacial surgery, going through mistakes I have made and the ways to avoid them in a primary care setting where the support may be minimal. I am sharing what I call "tricks of the trade" - ideas and concepts that have crystallised out of teaching received, and experience gained, by me.

My hope in writing this book is to simplify and debunk common oral surgical procedures, and increase your confidence in managing patients who require oral surgical intervention. I ask you to read it with an open mind and without any prejudice.

Dr Abdul Dalghous

1 Introduction

The extraction of teeth remains an essential part of both the art and the science of dentistry despite the enormous progress in the prevention of dental disease made during the last 30 years. It is one of the most common procedures practised daily in general dentistry.

With modern conservative dentistry, more and more people retain their teeth into later life. This means we see older patients who have more complicated medical histories and tougher, more brittle, less flexible bone than the young. Thus, the difficulty and complexity of extraction procedures is increasing with the average age of our patients.

Tooth extraction not only depends on the experience of the surgeon, but more importantly on their calm, reassuring manner while explaining the procedure to the usually anxious patient. It also depends on their ability to empathise with patients and the way they perceive the problem.

The dangers of minor oral surgery have been grossly exaggerated. In fact most of the fears experienced have little foundation. Excluding general anaesthesia, minor oral surgery with or without sedation is a remarkably safe undertaking.

The purpose of this book is to provide the general dentist with specific information about oral surgery procedures that are performed daily in primary care settings. Also, to pass on my vast experience in oral surgery to junior dentists and dentists with a special interest in oral surgery.

The book also aims to demystify the myths in oral surgery, and make teeth extraction fun rather than a challenge for the general dentist. One of the reasons for writing this book is to help and guide newly qualified dentists and general dentists working in primary care in order to build their confidence so that they will be able to risk assess and manage patients who need teeth extraction and other common oral surgical procedures. Also, they will learn practical skills to achieve anaesthesia and be able to deal with day-to-day patients requiring extractions or management of common acute dental infections. It will teach them how to achieve profound dental anaesthesia first time every time.

The ability of a general dentist to perform common oral surgical procedures is based on several factors. Some dentists have a great interest in surgery, while others have very little interest. Some dentists have had hospital or other postgraduate training or experience, others may not have had the opportunity. Some dentists work in practices or even areas that have little or no support from a specialist, which makes simple and complex oral surgery mandatory in their practices. Currently, it is accepted that regardless of who performs dental procedures, be they a dentist or a specialist, the standards of care are the same. If a general dentist wants to include the removal of third molars in his or her practice, he or she will usually need more training than that provided in dental school.

Just having the desire to do this procedure will not, in and of itself, qualify a person. The best thing a general dentist can do is to first obtain additional training. Surgical expertise is improved by taking postgraduate courses.

The clinician then learns to diagnose the less complicated procedures and carries them out under supervision until they are performed well. Therefore, the dentist has a greater responsibility to acquire training and knowledge if he or she expects to do more complex procedures. This responsibility includes not only receiving instruction in step-by-step surgical techniques, but also the medical management of such patients and any complications that might arise.

In my opinion, with the right exposure and training, every qualified dentist should have the skills and ability to assess, manage and extract simple to moderately difficult teeth. They should know how to avoid and deal with complications should they arise, and safely manage acute dentofacial infections. This will ensure that NHS patient waiting time is reduced, dentists maintain and improve their surgical skills, and if they work from private practice they keep their patients and income to themselves.

It is not uncommon to be faced with one of your loyal private patients who might be in severe pain from his or her infected or symptomatic tooth, but you say to them, "Sorry I can do a filling, perhaps whiten your teeth and make your teeth beautiful, but unfortunately I am not good enough to extract your infected tooth and get you out of pain. I will have to refer you to another dentist or a specialist or even the hospital where you may have to wait for a few hours, if not days or weeks, to be treated." That patient could be a pregnant lady in her last trimester, or a frail old lady with no one to look after her or even transport her to the hospital.

You can improve your surgical knowledge and gain enough skills to enable you to avoid the above scenario by reading and understanding this book, in addition to basic oral surgery books. You should also attend short practical and didactic hands-on courses on pigs' heads provided by a specialist or a consultant oral surgeon, or one of the courses that I run here under the auspices of Yorkshire Dental Suite (YDS) Academy. These are followed by attending a few clinical one-to-one training sessions on real patients, where you will have the opportunity to learn how to assess the difficulty of extraction, learn how to achieve profound anaesthesia, and perform simple as well as difficult extractions under supervision. In my opinion combining all of the above is invaluable.

I must say that I realise that writing this book is a risk for me and my reputation. There are certain people in the world, including some in the dental community, who may be very critical of my work. I used to be overly concerned about those critics' opinions. This book is different to most other oral surgery books which usually quote and repeat what is said and written by other authors and collate it in a book. I am literally writing down in simple words what I have practiced and preached every day over the last 30 years in the field of oral and maxillofacial surgery.

Warning: this book is not for students, and in fact if a student reads it they may not pass their exam. Also, it is not for faint-hearted and close-minded practitioners.

I must also mention that this book is not in any way a replacement of the recommended textbooks but as an adjunct. I will teach you all "the nuts and bolts" in oral surgery and the tricks I have learnt over more than 30 years. I have taken out tens of thousands of decayed teeth, broken roots and wisdom teeth in primary and secondary care settings under local anaesthetic (LA), intravenous (IV) sedation and general anaesthesia (GA) and I will teach you what works in my hands! I will tell you all the mistakes I have made, or seen done, and how to avoid them.

I will tell you the stuff they don't teach you at dental school (the taboo!), and I will teach you what to do, when to do it, and most importantly what not to do.

I am a massive advocate of performing a risk assessment in oral surgery. If you understand and practice the risk assessment that I am going to teach you then you should be able to deal efficiently with most, if not all, oral surgical cases that attend your practice.

The aim is to teach you risk assessment that, if applied correctly, assures that patient management will be swift, successful and complication-free for both the patient and the practitioner. It will save you time and money, make you even more money, and most importantly build you an excellent reputation and help your dentistry business to flourish. This book attempts to demystify techniques for local anaesthesia, teeth extraction and oral surgery.

I recommend this book to all who wish to learn all there is to know about the extraction of teeth in the young and the elderly, and I do so without hesitation or reservation. It is not just a book to read in your dental library – it is a book for everyday use!

I have included some thoughts and techniques that I would describe as tricks of the trade; ideas and concepts that have crystallised out of the teaching received and experience gained by me, and my hope is that newly qualified dentists with minimum experience in oral surgery will find something of value within these pages.

It summarises my experience which spans over 30 years in the field of oral and maxillofacial surgery. I have tried to make it simple, safe, exciting, practical, and not necessarily evidence based.

I guarantee that if you study, practice and master what is in this book, you will have no problem taking teeth out safely for any patient at any time of any day.

I hate theory-spewers. The people who publish crap that sounds great, but they don't practise it and have no idea if it works. This is different. This is real. The purpose of this book is simple - to give YOU all the tools you need to succeed in oral surgery. It's crucial to understand that the following tips, insights, and secrets can, and should, be applicable to you.

2 The oral surgery patient journey

It is important to plan a "journey" that is safe, efficient and enjoyable to both patient and surgeon. In a primary care setting, this journey normally begins with a patient seeking advice either from the practice website or through a telephone conversation with the front of house team. On arrival for a pre-booked appointment it is important to meet and greet the patient in a non-surgical setting, build a rapport with them and get to know their concerns and worries. Next comes escorting the patient through to the treatment room and conducting a thorough systematic examination and any necessary investigations. Once a diagnosis of the problem is reached, it is important to go through options, the pros and cons of each option, and obtain a valid informed consent. Finally, the patient should be booked in for the treatment. Before leaving they should be given an information leaflet which contains a phone number and an email address in case they need any further information or have questions (sometimes patients forget to ask during the consultation).

I always try to avoid same day extractions except in certain situations or emergencies. For example, if a patient is in severe pain or has a surgical emergency such as a severe dental abscess, or if they have travelled a long way, then as long as they understand fully what is involved I will carry out the treatment on the day of the consultation.

When a patient returns for treatment, my front of house team welcomes them, greets them with their name, and updates and confirms their details. I then make sure to personally greet them by their name, go through the consent again (remember consent is a continuous process) and answer any queries that may have arisen since the last time I saw them. I check that their details haven't changed, update their medical history (PMH) for any changes, make sure they have had their regular medications and a light meal (if not, I give them some food and drink while I am chatting with them). My assistant and I make sure that the treatment room is ready for the procedure, with all the necessary surgical equipment and local anaesthetic in place. I always make sure I have a surgical kit ready even for a simple extraction. I then discuss and confirm the plan with my assistant, and confirm that the treatment is what the patient has signed and consented to.

I always make sure my treatment room smells nice (I burn incense sticks in the room) and that it is clean and tidy. I also ask the patient for their choice of music to listen to. This makes them more relaxed and shows attention to detail and personalised care.

Once the patient is sitting comfortably in the dental chair (not crossing their legs, as that may impede the venous return from the legs to the heart and may precipitate blood clots), I double-check and confirm the tooth to be extracted (with nurse, patient, radiograph, consent and referral letter). Once I decide the LA technique, I make sure I give enough local anaesthetic - preferably using two different types of LA (more on this later). Once I administer the local anaesthetic, I do not poke the mucosa or the gum with a sharp probe and ask the patient if they feel anything sharp (as they teach you in dental school) to check for effective anaesthesia.

Be confident and positive, as a patient can sense your lack of confidence and you may lose their cooperation. Instead, I apply pressure to the patient's shoulder with my hand and advise them that this is the pressure they are going to feel during the extraction as I "push teeth out" and this is normal. However, I assure them that if they feel anything sharp at any time then they can raise their hand (on the side of the assistant) and I will stop immediately and possibly give them more LA if required.

I never send the patient back to the client lounge to wait for the local anaesthetic to work. This is mainly for two reasons. Firstly, and most importantly, is in case they have a reaction to the anaesthetic - be this due to toxicity or allergy - and secondly, the anaesthetic I use (Articaine) works within seconds.

Once the planned surgical procedure is completed, I place a damp gauze on the extraction site and ask the patient to bite down for 3-5 minutes (my nurse can go through after-care instructions while I write the patient's notes at this stage). I then check for haemostasis under a good light and discard the gauze in the clinical waste bin. I do not send the patient home with a gauze in their mouth. I give the patient a small take away bag containing extra sterile gauze and written instructions containing the practice contact number and out of hours emergency number. The front of house team will always call the patient (care call) after 24-48 hours to make sure they are OK. Patients do appreciate this after-care phone call.

3 The new oral surgery patient

A patient comes to see you for three main reasons: diagnostic purposes, treatment or reassurance, or a combination of these factors.

A clinical examination comprises three components: the history, the examination, and the explanation, where the dentist discusses the nature and implications of the clinical findings.

There is nothing more important than taking a full history and performing a thorough, systematic clinical examination of the patient to be able to establish a rapport, reach a diagnosis, and design a correct treatment plan. For this, sufficient time should be allowed, and an accurate clinical record should be ensured. Recording of negative findings is as important as positive ones.

To be a great surgeon you must be a great physician.

Unfortunately, many practising dentists nowadays are quite poor at taking patient history and performing a thorough head and neck examination. In my opinion, this is mainly due to lack of time, knowledge, and reliance on technology. Some dentists don't even look at the patient but instead they only look at their teeth!

They may miss obvious and important clinical features which may diagnose underlying disease or even oral cancer (eg, a patient with an obvious large midline neck lump may indicate thyrotoxicosis which may complicate treatment). I believe that changes in oral mucosa can give indications to the patient's general health and disease (the mouth is the gateway to the body). For example, diagnosis of anaemia, vitamin deficiency or even immune deficiency can be diagnosed from oral cavity examination (colour of tongue, thrush etc).

1. History

Make sure you identify the correct patient (some patients have the same name and even the same date of birth!), establish a rapport to make the patient feel at ease, introduce your team (nurse), and ensure the patient is sitting comfortably in the dental chair.

Be friendly but professional, and make the patient feel like he or she is the most important person in the room. Remember - not many people want to sit in a dental chair!

Take a full history of the patient's complaint (in their own words), and ensure medical, dental, and social history is completed. Ask specifically for any allergies to penicillin, latex, nuts and their severity (anaphylaxis/rash/sickness/diarrhoea?). If they have a history of osteoarthritis (OA), osteoporosis or cancer, ask specifically for any bisphospho-nate intake as some patients may think it's not important and may not volunteer the information. I recall one lady recently who was referred to me by her dentist with regards to a non-healing socket (Figure 3.1) just over a year post-extraction. To me it looked like MRONJ and when I specifically asked her whether she had taken alendronic acid in the past she said yes, and it was intravenously too.

She never gave this information to her caring dentist, nor mentioned it when she filled in her medical history form (both at her dentist and at my practice).

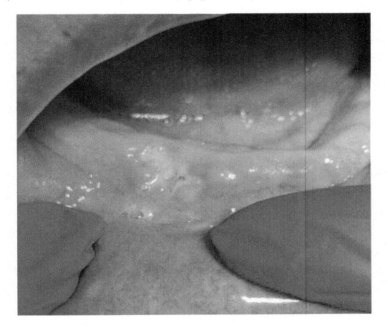

Figure 3.1 MRONJ post-extraction

2. Examination

From the moment the patient enters the surgery he or she should be carefully observed for signs of physical or psychological disease which may show in gait, the carriage, the general manner, or the relationship between parent and child.

In general, the principle of examination is "eyes first, then hands", not both together.

Examination can be divided into extraoral and intraoral:

A. Extraoral examination

Here, look for any facial asymmetry (swelling), skin colour (pale, red and shiny), facial muscle movements, cranial nerves especially the trigeminal (V) and the facial (VII), examine the lips for fissuring, enlargement (Crohn's, orofacial granulomatosis) or maceration of the corners of the mouth (candidiasis).

Examine the eyes. For example, pale conjunctiva may indicate anaemia, yellow sclera as in jaundice, or blue sclera as in osteogenesis/dentinogenesis imperfecta.

Stand behind the patient and ask them to flex their head forward to relax their neck muscles. Palpate the head and neck lymph nodes, in particular the parotid, submandibular and cervical (tenderness, enlargement, consistency, mobility). This is very important especially in high-risk patients (high tobacco and alcohol consumption or history of cancer).

Examine for tone and tenderness of facial muscles, assess and measure mouth opening (use a ruler or your fingers), TMJ looking for tenderness, locking, clicking, grating and range of movements.

B. Intraoral examination

Be systematic and examine lips (ulcers, fissure, or lumps), cheeks, floor of mouth, tongue (dorsal, ventral and especially posterior and lateral margins), soft and hard palate, and oropharynx (depress tongue with a mirror and ask patient to say 'Ah').

Look actively for any signs of sinister disease especially in high risk areas in high risk patients (indurated ulcer, red lesion, white patch, lump). If you find any lump then find out if it is hard (bone), firm (like cartilage in the tip of the nose) soft (fat), or fluctuant (fluid or pus).

If you find an ulcer then note down the site, size, shape, number, tenderness, induration or fixation.

Examine the parotid glands and Stensen's ducts opening (don't confuse it with a lump or polyp) and make sure there is free flow of saliva from the duct opening. Perform bimanual palpation of the submandibular salivary glands and check for tenderness and consistency.

Only then examine the teeth and periodontal tissues and then pay special attention to the patient's problem (carious tooth that may be tender to percussion, loose tooth, draining sinus, broken tooth, impacted tooth etc).

C. Special investigations

After the above is completed and a differential diagnosis is made, the need for further investigations should be considered. Always ask yourself, "Is it going to change my diagnosis or management? Will it help in explanation and consenting of the patient?" There is no such thing as routine radiograph or routine blood test. Each investigation must be justified.

D. Diagnosis

You must then make the correct diagnosis. If you are in any doubt, consult your colleagues and work as a team. Do not be shy in asking your senior colleagues for help. Incorrect diagnosis means incorrect treatment. Incorrect treatment means unhappy patients. Patients need their problem sorted as quickly as possible with the least risk and minimal inconvenience.

4 Indications for teeth extractions

Teeth may need to be removed due to various reasons. The tooth itself may be diseased or in the wrong place, or it may be involved in a disease involving the surrounding tissues. Most common examples are outlined below.

1. Unrestorable caries

If the tooth can't be restored due to extensive caries, or due to financial reasons, then extraction may be the only option, especially if the tooth is symptomatic or infected.

2. Sepsis

This could be chronic or acute, for example an acute dental abscess with cellulitis.

3. Advanced periodontal disease

If the tooth/teeth are affected with severe periodontal disease, then the affected teeth may have to be extracted to save the remaining teeth and improve the patient's oral and general health.

4. Failed root canal treatment (RCT)

If a repeat RCT, with or without radicular surgery, is not an option due to poor prognosis or financial reasons, or it has been tried and failed, then extraction may be the only option.

5. Trauma

Severely broken or subluxated teeth that can't be saved by restorative means may have to be extracted.

6. Orthodontic treatment

The most common teeth to be extracted as part of orthodontic treatment are first premolars, impacted canines, or retained baby teeth. This is to create space for moving misaligned teeth, correcting the occlusion, and improving aesthetics and oral health.

7. Pathology (cyst/tumours) (Figure 4.1) or part of tumour resection or cyst removal

8. Prophylactic extraction prior to radiotherapy (RT) to the head and neck or chemotherapy (CT)

Teeth with poor or questionable prognosis are sometimes extracted prior to starting radiotherapy or anti-resorptive therapy (bisphosphonate) to prevent complications (osteoradionecrosis (ORN) and medication related osteonecrosis of the jawbone (MRONJ)).

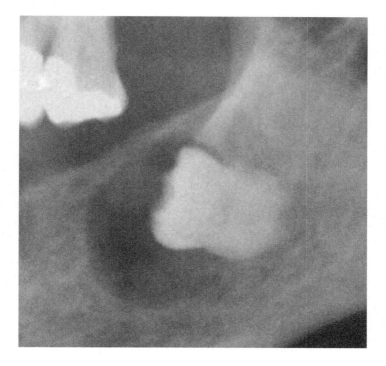

Figure 4.1 Dentigerous cyst associated with impacted LL8

9. Teeth in line of a jaw fracture if they interfere with fracture reduction and/or fixation

For example, impacted or partially erupted lower wisdom teeth associated with mandibular angle fracture.

10. Malposed and impacted teeth. For example, partially erupted symptomatic wisdom teeth

11. Extraction of retained baby teeth to create space for permanent teeth or placement of dental implant

5 Contraindications for teeth extractions

There are NO absolute contraindications for teeth extractions. However, there are a few situations and conditions where extra care or precautions should be taken and sometimes liaison with a specialist or physician is recommended.

I would not extract a tooth for a haemophiliac or leukaemia patient with severe liver or kidney disease in a primary care setting. They are at risk of uncontrolled post-extraction bleeding and therefore may need factor replacement or specialist care which can only be given in the hospital. I would also avoid extraction for a patient who is taking, or who has had, IV bisphosphonate therapy or radiotherapy for the head and neck.

In case of concern, it is prudent to discuss potential problems with the patient's physician. It must, however, be remembered that advice once sought must be taken, and will always tend to err on the side of caution. Each case should be assessed individually, and the pros and cons of the procedure should be discussed in detail with the patient before a decision can be made.

For example, in the case of pregnant ladies it is better to perform elective treatments in the mid trimester. However, emergency treatment can be performed at any time with caution. Treatment in the first few weeks of pregnancy can be complicated due to physiological body and mood changes. For example, severe sickness and gag reflex can make administration of LA or extraction of posterior teeth difficult, especially in nervous patients where intravenous sedation is contraindicated. Also, all types of medications including antibiotics should be avoided as it may affect the development of the foetus. Extraction in late pregnancy can be complicated by poor patient positioning, difficult access, and the potential of supine hypotension syndrome if a patient with a gravid uterus is laid back for a long time.

6 Complications of teeth extractions

Extraction of teeth is one of the most performed procedures in primary and secondary care clinics. It stands to reason that most of the complications we see are related to oral surgery. These can be common or rare and can occur before, during or after treatment. Nevertheless, with careful treatment planning and adherence to good surgical techniques and principles, surgeons can minimise the frequency of complications. In addition, early recognition and proper management can help to improve the outcome of procedures. Because complications are a risk and potential sequelae of any surgery, it is imperative that surgeons notify patients of them while obtaining informed consent. Unfortunately, complications can occur even when the surgeon adheres to good surgical principles. Variations in anatomy and the patient's response to healing can result in complications even when the surgeon executes the surgical procedure within the standard of care.

Every practising dentist should be able to recognise and manage extraction complications.

To be an amazing and caring oral surgeon, you should be able to prevent and deal with any potential extraction complications. It does not mean you should have the skills of a specialist surgeon from the get-go, but you should be able to predict and manage oral surgery complications. Management may simply mean knowing your limitations (skills or tools), and when and who to refer the patient to for safe treatment.

Oral surgery produces tissue damage and patient morbidity, therefore every operation must be justified by weighing the benefits against the risks. The purpose must be either elimination of disease, prevention of disease, improvement of function, or aesthetics.

For example, removal of an asymptomatic retained root inflicts certain surgical damage and in my opinion is not justified by the hypothetical risk of future infection.

Overestimation of difficulty leads to relief and gratitude, while underestimation leads to embarrassment at least, and distress and litigation at worst.

Thorough planning and preparation are the keys to successful surgery. "If you fail to prepare then you prepare to fail". Efficiency wins and maintains patients' confidence and cooperation. Difficulties arise more often from lack of planning, or forethought, than from any lack of knowledge or manual skills.

Complications in oral surgery are sometimes inevitable. Always expect them, pre-warn your patient about them, and be prepared to deal with them should they arise.

Whilst the risk of certain adverse events can be minimised with forethought at the assessment stage (risk assessment) and careful execution of the surgery, some of the problems that arise are totally unpredictable.

In my opinion, if you do not know how, or do not have the ability or the support from colleagues, to manage extraction complications, then maybe you are not qualified for the procedure. The best management of complications is to prevent them in the first place. Most common complications that I have come across during my last 30 years in oral surgery can be broadly divided into pre-operative, intra-operative and post-operative as follows:

1. Pre-operative complications include difficulty in access, poor patient cooperation (related to patient medical history), and difficulty in achieving anaesthesia.

2. Intra-operative complications include failure to complete an extraction, fracture of the tooth, damage to other teeth, loss of tooth/roots, OACs, soft tissue trauma, damage to nerves, fractures of the alveolus/mandible, and dislocation of the TMJ.

3. Post-operative complications include haemorrhage, excessive pain, swelling, dry socket, infection, ORN, MRONJ, trismus, and surgical emphysema.

Good technique and comprehensive clinical and radiographic assessment will minimise many of these complications.

A. Pre-operative complications

1. Difficult access to surgical site

Limitation of mouth opening (trismus) can be due to acute dentoalveolar infection, TMJ dysfunction, microstomia, kyphosis, parkinsonism or severe learning disability. If you can't access the surgical site adequately then it is hard or impossible to complete the surgery or achieve adequate anaesthesia even in the easy straightforward cases. These cases should be identified early on during the assessment stage. For these patients consider IV sedation or referral to hospital for treatment under general anaesthetic. If the trismus is due to infection, then postpone the treatment if possible until the infection is resolved with antibiotics, with or without drainage of the abscess.

2. Poor patient cooperation

A lack of patient cooperation will be a barrier to effective extractions. This could be due to young age or a previous bad experience at the dentist. Prior to commencing any extraction, a discussion and judgement should be made to determine whether the patient will likely tolerate the procedure under local anaesthetic only, or whether IV sedation or referral to the hospital for treatment with GA is necessary.

3. Failure to achieve LA

There is absolutely no reason for this to ever happen. It is frustrating when it happens, and most of us have experienced it at some stage of our career. Failure to achieve adequate anaesthesia for the inferior dental nerve (IDN) is not uncommon in the hands of newly qualified and less experienced clinicians. The main reason in my opinion is due to not giving enough anaesthetic in the right place (see later LA section).

4. Complications related to medical conditions

These include patients who are ASAII or above, or patients taking medications including anticoagulants, antiplatelets, bisphosphonate, etc. These patients should be identified early on, and arrangements should be made for their safe treatment.

B. Intra-operative complications

1. Fracture of the LA needle

This is extremely unlikely with modern disposable needles. However, it happened to me while I was teaching live on one of our implant courses when I accidentally used an UltraSafe Plus syringe instead of using an UltraSafe Twist extra short LA cartridge (not compatible). It snapped while I was giving palatal infiltration and I lost sight of the needle as it dived into the posterior fatty part of the palatal mucosa. Of course, I kept cool and was still able to feel it and pick it out with fine mosquito forceps.

Avoid bending the needle and making sudden changes in the direction of the needle while it is deep in tissue (eg, IDN block) and never insert the needle up to the hub (weakest point) so it is easy to retrieve if it breaks. Avoid using an extra short fine needle in patients with uncontrolled movements as it may lead to needle breakage. In this case it is best to use a longer needle as a sudden movement of the patient while the needle is deep in the tissue may cause the needle to break.

2. Extraction of the wrong tooth

This has never happened to me, even after extraction of hundreds of thousands of teeth over the years, and it should never happen to anyone as it is fully preventable. It is devastating when it happens. Unfortunately, it is not uncommon and is under-reported, therefore full attention must always be practised. I saw a patient while I was working at a hospital who was on intravenous alendronic acid (Fosamax) for treatment of cancer. The wrong tooth had been extracted by a trainee (he also had the correct tooth extracted too)! This is a common source of litigation and is indefensible. It is most commonly due to the use of a different teeth numbering system (if a referral), difference in mounting of radiographs, or simply operator fatigue, complacency and lack of attention. Extraction of the wrong tooth can also happen to the wrong patient. Therefore, it is paramount to confirm the correct patient at the reception desk and by the surgeon during the consenting process. Confirm by asking the patient's name, address and date of birth. It is not uncommon for two different patients to have the same name and sometimes the same date of birth! When you get the patient into your surgery always double check their identity and triple check the tooth to be extracted. Confirm with the patient, radiograph, team and the referring dentist. Especially with referrals, the referring dentist may have requested extraction of the wrong tooth which did happen with a patient who was referred to me. When I called the dentist, he agreed with me and apologised, and no harm was done.

During the extraction, stay focused and do not get distracted. Never ever have a conversation with your nurse or staff about anything not related to your patient when your patient is in the dental chair.

Should an error occur, the patient must be informed, and the surgeon must proceed to extract the right tooth to complete the operation. A decision then must be made whether to reimplant the wrongly extracted tooth immediately and splint it, or to accept the situation.

3. Failure to move a tooth

Find out why the tooth is not moving and never apply excessive force. Stay calm, put the forceps down and take a deep breath. Examine the buccal plate thickness. The thicker the plate the harder it is to mobilise a tooth. Take a radiograph and assess the anatomy, bone thickness and quality. Check for hypercementosis or ankylosis (if you can't see the lamina dura around the roots that means the roots are more likely to be ankylosed) and the number, size and shape of roots. If in any doubt, then consider surgical extraction as this may be quicker and less destructive to hard and soft tissues (section the tooth and even raise a flap if necessary).

In general, the way I extract a tooth, I stand on the right of the patient to remove the teeth on the right side and on the left to remove the teeth on the left side (ie, on the same side of the tooth to be extracted). However, I stand on the right side for extraction of all the upper teeth. I extend my arm fully and apply force from my shoulder rather than my wrist to move the tooth. This enables me to apply more force and avoid damage to my wrist. I know of at least one dentist who broke his wrist while taking a tooth out (you know who you are)!

Access to the maxillary third molar can be difficult even in a patient with no restriction of mouth opening. This is because when the patient fully opens, the coronoid process moves into the area of the maxillary third and second molars, limiting instrumentation access. Access into this area can be improved by having the patient close slightly and move the mandible laterally to the side of the tooth to be extracted. This will move the coronoid process away from the surgical site and improve access.

4. Fracture of a tooth/root

This may be due to extensive caries, heavy restoration, long divergent roots, dense bone, or wrong extraction technique. Very thick buccal plates and the presence of bony exostosis around the teeth to be extracted may prevent bone expansion and increase the risk of tooth fracture. In these cases, consider surgical extraction to ensure a more predictable outcome. It is not uncommon, especially if you grab the crown of the tooth rather than the root, use excessive force, or use the wrong extraction forceps. To avoid this mishap, never hold the crown but always engage the roots with the correct forceps (Figure 6.1).

Some teeth are expected to break, and they should have been identified during the risk assessment. A plan should be designed to remove them surgically.

Avoid the tendency to pull the tooth buccally to minimise the chances of forceps' peaks slipping and holding the crown instead. So, remember 'push teeth out' (not pull). Moreover, move the tooth in all directions even in multirooted teeth (forget what the textbooks say) provided you use slow, steady, and controlled movements maintaining apical pressure all the time. Moving the tooth should be slow, steady, and purposeful and not a series of short, jerky, shaking gestures which are both ineffective and unpleasant for the patient. Stick to this and you are less likely to break any tooth (of course if your risk assessment is sound).

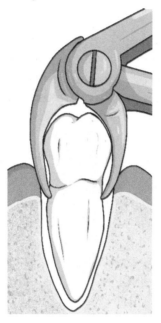

Figure 6.1 Note the beaks are holding the root not the crown

If the tooth is broken, then a decision must be made whether to leave or remove the residual root. This requires anticipating whether the root fragment will remain asymptomatic or whether it will become infected and cause pain (non-infected roots do not cause pain), perhaps lead to an abscess and a discharging sinus, develop a cyst, or interfere with a denture or implant placement or orthodontic tooth movement. The risks of continued, more aggressive attempts at retrieval of the root tip might outweigh the benefits. If, however, the root breaks after the tooth has become mobile, then it should be removed as it will almost certainly become infected and cause pain.

5. Damage to adjacent teeth

This mishap can be caused by careless application of the elevator or forceps. Subluxation of adjacent teeth is most common when extracting the first molar causing subluxation or damage to the premolar, as the premolar is the weakest link here. I see this a lot with junior trainees as they focus on luxating the tooth without paying attention to the adjacent tooth. It is also common with crowded lower anterior teeth where the space is very limited even for the smallest extraction forceps, and if care is not taken by doing surgical extraction, then subluxation of adjacent teeth may happen.

The watching fingers of the supporting hand can assist in preventing this by feeling that the forceps are in a good position and detecting even slight movements in adjacent teeth. I also tell my assistant to keep an eye open and to stop me immediately if she notices that the wrong tooth is moving.

Luxators and elevators are great tools, but they must be used safely and correctly and only when indicated (do not use them routinely).

Fracture of restorations of an adjacent tooth, especially teeth restored with crowns, can also happen so make sure you hold the correct tooth without touching the crown of the adjacent tooth. One important aspect is if the adjacent teeth have fillings, crowns or veneers, then one way of minimising the risk of damage during extraction is to cut into the mesial and distal surfaces of the tooth to be extracted to create room for tooth movement and avoid damage to restorations. For this it is best to use a diamond bur on a turbine handpiece.

Never lean on a tooth or touch restoration of adjacent teeth during extraction. Of course, always pre-warn patients of this small risk.

Never use adjacent teeth as a fulcrum unless they too are to be extracted (for example lower or upper clearance).

Move the tooth slowly in all directions to allow the alveolar bone to expand, making sure you apply apical pressure all the time.

6. Damage to antagonist teeth

If you use excessive pulling force in the opposite direction you may damage the opposite tooth, fillings or crowns. Damage can happen when drawing a tooth from its socket without sufficient control and it may bang against the upper teeth. This is more common in the extraction of lower teeth as they require more vertical traction. Remember, use controlled force during extraction and do not rush.

7. Osseous injuries and maxillary tuberosity fracture

Dentoalveolar and/or maxillary tuberosity fracture is not uncommon and sometimes unavoidable, usually without any consequences. Alveolar bone fracture is most common with the extraction of upper anterior teeth, upper molars and lower anterior teeth. Fracture of the antral floor is also common and may lead to oroantral communication (more later).

Risk factors include divergent, bulbous and hypercementosed roots, thick buccal cortical plates, old age (reduced bone elasticity), and bone diseases such as osteogenesis imperfecta.

You should be able to tell from your risk assessment if tuberosity fracture is likely to happen and what steps you should be taking to avoid it. To reduce the risk of this complication, avoid using a large elevator or luxator to push teeth distally if they are fully erupted. If they are, then try to use forceps and not an elevator. Never use a Coupland or Cryer elevator to force the tooth out as this will most likely cause a dentoalveolar/tuberosity fracture. If there is no movement then find out why and consider surgical extraction. If you break the tuberosity and the tooth is still attached with palatal laceration, then do not panic.

Fracture of a maxillary tuberosity is common and usually goes unnoticed. However, fracture of a large part of the tuberosity can be quite serious and troublesome to patient and surgeon. It is most common if the tooth is ankylosed or with strong long roots and if a large elevator (Coupland or Cryer) was applied to push the tooth distally. Never use any elevator other than a Warwick James to mobilise the upper wisdom tooth, and as soon as the tooth is loose then hold it with suitable forceps (usually bayonet) and deliver it buccally. If you see blanching or tearing of the palate while elevating upper 8 then stop immediately as that may be a sign of tuberosity breaking (Figures 6.2 and 6.3).

Management of broken tuberosity is as follows: If small, remove the fractured bone fragment with the tooth. If the tooth (usually upper 8) is very loose, then gently detach it from the mucosa, take it out and achieve a primary closure (Figure 6.4).

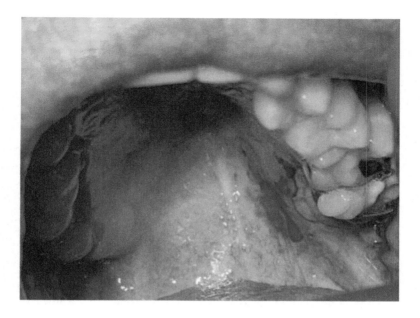

Figure 6.2 Tear of palatal mucosa

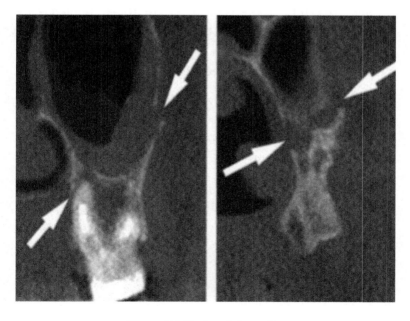

Figure 6.3 Broken tuberosity

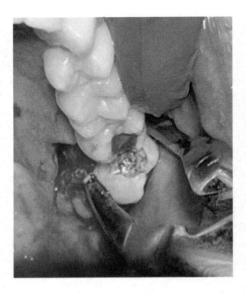

Figure 6.4 Broken tuberosity with tooth still attached to the mucosa

If the bone fragment is attached to the periosteum, dissect off the tooth. If the tooth is loose and unable to detach from the mucosa, then abandon the extraction and splint it to the adjacent teeth (flexi wire and composite) and defer the extraction for at least 6-8 weeks.

If the tooth must be removed due to pain or infection, then grasp the tooth with forceps and dissect the mucosa off with a sharp periosteal elevator or a fine luxator until the tooth, with or without the broken bone, is completely removed.

Every effort should be made to avoid tearing the palatal mucosa. On rare occasions, you may even have to raise the buccal flap and section the bone to free the tooth.

8. Oroantral communication (OAC)

OAC should be expected following any extractions of upper teeth from upper premolars to 3rd molar and the patient should be consented about the small risk of OAC. Most OAC have no consequences and go unnoticed. However, a small proportion may cause complications if untreated promptly. Always make sure you have a surgical tray before you extract upper molars especially in cases where the possibility of OAC is high (identified from your risk assessment).

If you break a root and you decide to remove it, then always have a low threshold for raising a flap (three-sided flap), removing bone and sectioning the tooth or root to minimise damage to alveolar bone and tearing of the soft tissue. Also, avoid using the luxator or elevator parallel to the long axis of the root but instead use it perpendicular and push the root downward rather than apically to avoid displacement of the tooth/roots into the sinus.

Small oroantral communication (less than 5mm) probably happens after the extraction of any upper molar and even premolar teeth. However, it recovers spontaneously in most cases. I never actively check for OAC after extractions by asking the patient to blow their nose with their mouth open etc, or asking them to perform the "Valsalva manoeuvre" as there is a small risk that it may enlarge the hole, and a small OAC after a simple extraction usually heals without problems and goes unnoticed.

If you create a large OAC that needs immediate repair, then you will probably see it quite clearly (a hole in the sinus). Also, when you irrigate with saline to clean out the extraction socket you may see it coming out through the nose. It is much easier to treat the OAC rather than an established fistula. Any communication less than 7mm usually heals spontaneously without complications. A large OAC should be closed immediately or within two to three days to avoid sinus infection.

The best way to deal with OAC is to try and prevent it in the first place by careful assessment of the patient clinically (see risk assessment) and using appropriate radiograph (proximity to sinus and long strong divergent roots). If there is any suspicion then it is best to do a surgical extraction sectioning the roots and avoiding apical pressure when delivering the tooth.

Make sure you warn the patient not to forcefully blow their nose for at least a week and to keep their mouth open if sneezing becomes necessary.

9. Soft tissue injuries

These can be due to trauma as a result of the careless application of extraction forceps, elevator or luxator or the surgical bur or drill or even scalpel (poor operator control).

When you apply the forceps during extraction, always make sure you apply them lingually first for lower teeth as you may crush the lingual mucosa that may contain the nerve causing nerve damage or laceration and bleeding. Then engage the forceps' peaks buccally making sure not to grip the buccal mucosa either.

I remember one day at the end of a busy Friday, I agreed to extract LR8 for a colleague (midwife). The tooth was partially erupted and looked easy, so I decided to have a go without raising a flap. I managed to luxate after a few minutes and then when I applied the lower molar forceps to retrieve the tooth, I pulled a long strip of buccal alveolar mucosa almost to the lower first premolar area. Luckily, it was superficial. The mental nerve was not exposed, and I managed to suture it with very fine resorbable sutures. It took a few days to heal but was very painful for the patient (as painful as a large oral ulcer). Therefore, always do your proper risk assessment beforehand and never be complacent.

Damage to soft tissue can also be due to lack of attention when handling the delicate oral mucosa or inadequate access due to raising a small flap, excessive flap retraction, or the use of excessive force. Be careful not to crush the lower lip against the lower teeth during extraction of the upper teeth, especially if the lower lip is also anaesthetised (it happened to me a couple of times, painful for the patient and embarrassing for me!).

Thermal injury to lips or cheeks unfortunately can sometimes happen and is due to overheating of the shank of the surgical bur or worn bearing of the handpiece (also happened to me once). The surgeon cannot feel the rise in temperature until it is too late because surgical gloves provide thermal insulation. Also, if you use the handpiece straight after coming from the autoclave while still too hot it may cause a similar problem. Advise your assistant to keep an eye on soft tissue while you are using the surgical handpiece and to stop you immediately if the shaft unintentionally touches the soft tissue (Figure 6.5).

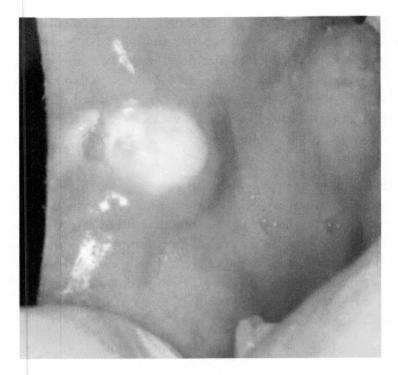

Figure 6.5 Lip laceration during the use of a surgical drill

10. Loss of tooth, root, or filling

Nothing is quite as unnerving to a dentist than realising that the tooth or root that is being extracted is no longer visible. If this happens, stop and alert the assistant. Conduct a systematic search and ask yourself:

1. is it in suction or the spittoon? (if it is, you are lucky!)

2. is it in the mouth/recent extraction sockets/under the tongue/floor of the mouth/oropharynx?

3. is it in the stomach or chest?

4. is it under the periosteum, particularly in the mandible where a flap has been raised? In this situation, a finger should be placed below the root and kept there to prevent it from going deeper. A flap may be raised to expose the root which can then be lifted out using a blunt hooked instrument. Never try to grasp it with forceps as if you miss then it may disappear into deeper spaces.

5. Maxillary anterior teeth or roots can accidentally be displaced into the floor of the nose or canine fossa whereas maxillary premolars and molars can be displaced into the maxillary sinus, infratemporal fossa and buccal space. Mandibular teeth or roots can be displaced into sublingual space, submandibular space, buccal space, parapharyngeal space or inferiorly into the inferior dental canal.

6. If not careful, distal movement of an impacted upper 8 may displace it into the soft tissue space behind the tuberosity of the maxilla to lie in the pterygomandibular space (Figure 6.6) or even in infratemporal fossa (Figure 6.7). Rare, but can be a very serious complication.

Displacement of a root into the sinus can be prevented if the following rules are followed:

1. Do not apply forceps to a root below the antrum unless there is sufficient exposure of the root to allow the forceps' blades to grasp the root securely under direct supervision.

2. Have a low threshold for leaving the apical third of maxillary molar palatal roots unless there is absolute indication for their removal.

In general, never be tempted to retrieve a root below the antrum by passing an instrument up into the socket. Instead, raise a three-sided flap and retrieve it from top down under direct vision.

If local measures to retrieve the root fail, then the patient should be referred to a specialist for exploration and root removal possibly via the Caldwell-Luc approach.

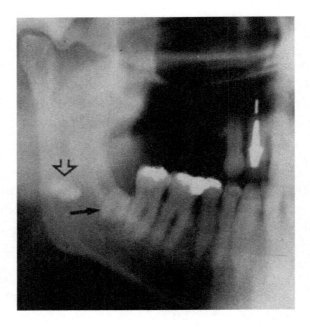

Figure 6.6 Pterygomandibular space

Swallowing of a tooth happened to one of my patients while I was extracting her lower wisdom tooth and it is not fun (I could not sleep that night until the tooth passed out the opposite end!). With careful assessment you can predict and prevent the likelihood of possible aspiration. I remember one patient in her late 50s. She was slightly obese, with a short neck, large strong masseters, thick buccal plate, and a heavily amalgam-filled and broken down UL7 with long splayed roots that were very close to the antrum. It was at the end of the day on a Friday. As soon as I applied forceps, I could see amalgam filling going down the oropharynx. It was very scary for a few seconds that felt like a few hours. Luckily, I had a good nurse who acted quickly to aspirate the fragment. I immediately sat the patient upright as quickly as possible, encouraged her to cough, and applied gentle blows to her back to help her cough and expel the fragments. I managed to complete the extraction successfully but believe me it was not a nice experience.

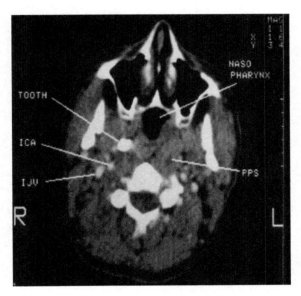

Figure 6.7 Infratemporal fossa

If a patient swallows a tooth, fillings or crowns, there is usually no cough or respiratory distress. In this case all you need to do is reassure the patient, document the incident, and advise the patient to watch for the tooth passing out from the other end in the following days (no need to send to A&E).

If a tooth or foreign object is aspirated (Figure 6.8), the patient will start coughing violently, resulting in respiratory distress and a drop in oxygen saturation. This is a surgical emergency and should be treated as choking. Immediate referral to hospital is necessary for further management which may be in the form of chest X-rays, bronchoscopy or even thoracotomy to save the patient's life. To prevent this serious complication, avoid laying the patient flat, be vigilant, use powerful suction and always ask the patient to breathe through their nose when you are about to extract the tooth or root to reduce the risk of inhalation.

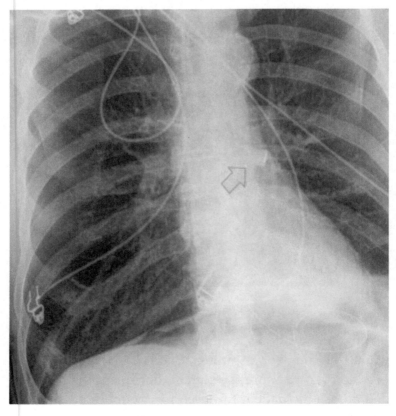

Figure 6.8 A swallowed tooth

11. TMJ damage (sometimes unavoidable in susceptible patients)

TMJ trauma can be caused due to excessive downward pressure or keeping the mouth wide open for too long, and may cause jaw dislocation or symptoms of myofascial pain dysfunction syndrome (MPDS). It is most seen in patients with a history of jaw dislocation or a prolonged surgical procedure. Make sure you support the lower jaw when applying force for extraction. Avoid the use of excessive force - which means you may have to section the tooth and the roots to make it easier to remove.

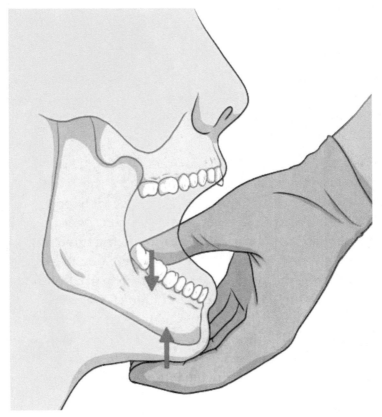

Figure 6.9 Reduction of dislocated lower jaw

12. Dislocation of the mandible

This is the dislodgement of the condyloid process from the glenoid fossa. This could be unilateral or bilateral and is due to excessive pressure on the mandible during extraction force and inadequate support to the mandible. If this happens during the extraction, it can be easily reduced by gentle manipulation (push the mandible downward and backward one side at a time). It is easier to reduce as soon as it happens before the muscles go into spasm (Figure 6.9).

13. Jaw fracture

This complication is rare. However, I did see it happen in the hospital following extraction of the upper first molar with the careless use of a number 3 Coupland's elevator where the whole dentoalveolar segment carrying the teeth broke off (the trainee registrar had tried to do the extraction quickly to impress me!).

Fracture of the mandible is extremely rare, therefore I do not consent my patient for it routinely for the extraction of lower wisdom teeth. However, I have seen it happen twice. Once was in a primary care setting where I got called by the dentist to confirm and manage the fractured angle of the mandible (Figure 6.10). It was purely due to excessive brutal force during the extraction of a partially erupted lower wisdom tooth where the dentist was forcing the tooth out with brute force in a rush rather than surgically removing it. The other case was in a hospital where a large dentigerous cyst, associated with an impacted lower wisdom tooth, was removed by a trainee registrar. A few days later the patient came back with a broken jaw.

Most common causes of jaw fractures are the use of excessive force during tooth extraction, excessive bone removal during surgery, atrophic mandible (Figure 6.11), osteolytic pathology-like cyst, chronic infection, osteomyelitis, tumour, and brittle bone diseases.

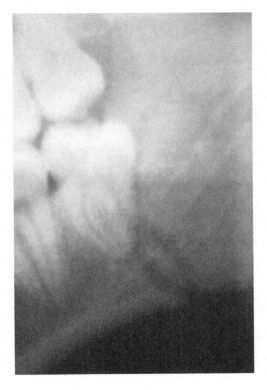

Figure 6.10 Fracture L angle of mandible

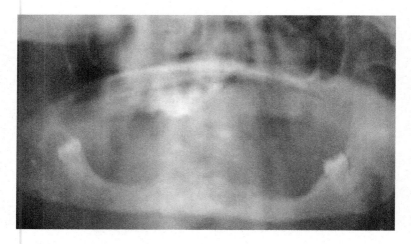

Figure 6.11 OPT showing old man with now symptomatic LL8 that needs SR (risk of jaw fracture)

C. Post-operative complications

1. Dry socket (alveolar osteitis)

This is the most common complication I see in my practice, especially following the extraction of difficult lower wisdom teeth. It is difficult to prevent but easy to manage.

Usually, the patient presents to the clinic two to three days following a difficult extraction. Signs and symptoms include severe pain at the extraction site radiating to the ear, accompanied by a bad smell and taste. There is no pus in a true dry socket (Figure 6.12).

Predisposing factors include lower molar extraction, traumatic extraction, a female on oral contraceptives, a history of dry sockets, smoking, poor oral hygiene, and excessive use of mouth wash following the extraction.

It is usually managed by reassurance and explanation of the condition, irrigation of the socket with saline, and lightly packing it with Alvogyl dressing. Repeated treatment may be necessary. Encourage the use of NSAIDs (non-steroidal anti-inflammatory drugs) and a simple analgesic plus warm salt water mouth rinse. Review if necessary. DO NOT anaesthetise and curettage the socket to encourage bleeding as this will cause more trauma and inflammation to the already inflamed socket.

If it does not heal within a few days, reconsider your diagnosis and exclude osteomyelitis or sinister disease (you may need to take an OPT).

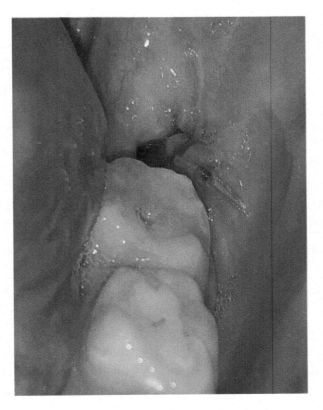

Figure 6.12 Dry socket

2. Infection

This is most commonly due to debris or a foreign body left in the extraction socket and is more common in immunocompromised patients. Common presentation includes swelling, pus discharge from or adjacent to the extraction socket, and lymphadenopathy. Treatment will be carried out depending on severity but may include drainage or antibiotics. If infection continues, progresses or becomes severe enough, it may spread to the bone, causing osteomyelitis. This is more likely in a patient who is immunocompromised or has other underlying medical problems.

3. Sensory nerve damage

This can be in the form of paraesthesia, which is spontaneous altered sensation that is not painful, dysaesthesia which is spontaneous altered sensation which is painful, hyperaesthesia which is excessive sensitivity to stimuli, hypoaesthesia which is decreased sensitivity to stimuli, anaesthesia which is no response to stimuli, or allodynia which is pain in response to normal non-painful stimuli.

It can be caused by a crush injury to the nerve due to poor flap design, the careless use of a surgical drill during osteotomy (if the drill slips and hits a nerve) or a blade while raising a mucoperiosteal flap. Rarely, it can be due to needle stick injury during LA administration. This will be identified if the patient reports any sharp shock-like pain during the injection. In this case the needle should be immediately withdrawn rather than continuing to inject as you have 'found the nerve'. Many injuries do recover, but they tend to take much longer than crush injuries.

Sensory nerve damage is a known complication associated with lower wisdom teeth extractions. However, with a proper risk assessment, careful surgery and appropriate radiographs, this should be minimal.

I do not see the use of a CBCT scan as necessary and OPT is more than enough for over 95% of cases. In a small number of cases, for example if there is a clear indication of IDN involvement, then CBCT may be considered to help planning of the procedure and patient consent.

4. Bleeding

Troublesome post-extraction bleeding is uncommon. After tooth extraction, it is normal for the area to bleed and then clot, generally within a few minutes. It is abnormal if the bleeding continues without clot formation or lasts beyond eight to 12 hours. This is known as post-extraction bleeding (PEB). Such bleeding incidents can cause distress for patients, who might need emergency dental visits and interventions. It can be caused by a variety of factors which are divided into local or systemic.

Local causes of bleeding include soft tissue and bone bleeding. Systemic causes include platelet problems, coagulation disorders or excessive fibrinolysis, and inherited or acquired problems (medication induced). There is a wide array of techniques suggested for the treatment of post-extraction bleeding, which include interventions aimed at both local and systemic causes.

Systemic factors can be excluded by taking a full and thorough patient PMH prior to the extraction. However, all bleeding sockets can be controlled locally using simple measures. First, you need to identify if it is bony or soft tissue bleeding and then treat accordingly. Apply pressure by placing a finger on each side of the alveolus to find the bleeding point. If bleeding stops then this indicates bleeding from soft tissue, and sutures may be placed across the socket (ideally horizontal mattress). Where pressure fails to arrest the haemorrhage, bleeding is from the bony socket, and this should be managed by placing a Whitehead's varnish pack in the socket, or bone wax. Alternatively, pack the socket with a haemostatic agent (Surgicel), suture, and apply pressure for 30 minutes. Keep reassuring the patient throughout and ask for help if you need to. Assess the patient's ABC and record vital signs including BP, pulse and O2 saturation.

Keep the patient under observation for at least an hour, give them fluid (sugary drink) and ensure the bleeding has stopped completely before they are discharged.

There are contradictory opinions on the discontinuation of antithrombotic medications. I do not normally interfere with patient medications, unless strongly advised by the patient's physician, as the prognosis of potential post-extraction bleeding that could result from antithrombotic continuation is better than the prognosis of a potential stroke or heart attack that could follow antithrombotic interruption.

It is important to note that it is not only the drugs that are important but also why the patient is taking them. My protocol for managing patients who are on anticoagulants (novel oral anticoagulant (NOAC) and warfarin) is as follows:

If they are on NOAC, then usually I do not interfere with their medication. If they are on warfarin, then I make sure I check INR within 48 hours, and if it is below 4 then you can proceed with the following precautions:

A. Utilise the first appointment of the day if possible

B. Ensure the patient has eaten and taken their usual medication

C. Check that a surgical tray and haemostatic agent is available

D. Give LA as needed (no contraindications for nerve block)

E. Avoid flap unless necessary

F. Always pack and suture the socket

G. Re-check haemostasis after 1 hour before the patient is discharged with verbal and written instructions

H. Always make a next day care call

5. Air (surgical) emphysema

This is a very rare but potentially fatal complication if not treated properly. It is usually due to air forced under pressure into connective tissues or facial planes, and is diagnosed with sudden onset facial swelling. There will be crepitus on palpation which differentiates it from surgical haematoma. To prevent this, avoid using a fast speed turbine handpiece for surgical extraction once a flap is raised and use a surgical handpiece instead. There should be spontaneous resolution within days, with or without antibiotics, but make sure you review the patient to ensure there is no infection. Note, however, it can lead to serious complications requiring hospitalisation.

6. Haematoma

This could be due to the needle accidentally injecting into a muscle or artery (eg, during IDN injection) and it should be differentiated from post-extraction infection. Management is usually by reassurance and close follow up.

7. Trismus

The most common cause of trismus following extraction is inflammatory oedema and swelling. Another common cause is intramuscular injection during IDN anaesthesia in which there is trauma to the medial pterygoid muscle, or penetration of small blood vessels and haematoma. Usually this will resolve within a few days to a few weeks with or without treatment.

8. Excessive pain

Pain can occur due to a traumatic or incomplete extraction, soft tissue trauma, exposed bone, infections or nerve damage. Management is through the identification and correction of the cause, and analgesics. Analgesia in the form of 1gm Paracetamol and 400mg Ibuprofen TDS is usually sufficient. Tramadol in my experience is not usually very effective for dental pain.

9. Swelling

A certain degree of swelling due to inflammatory oedema following the extraction is to be expected. The gentler in handling the tissues you are, the less post-operative swelling the patient will experience (handle the tissue gently as if you are handling a lady).

10. Osteomyelitis

This is very rare in healthy patients but should be excluded if the healing of the post-extraction socket is delayed. It is more common in the lower jaw than the upper, especially in patients with suppressed immunity or poor oral hygiene. Lower lip paraesthesia in the site of the extraction may differentiate it from a dry socket or simple infection. Take a radiograph which may reveal a moth-eaten appearance (sequestrum and involucrum). Treatment usually involves debridement and decortication of the dead bone, with or without antibiotics, and close follow up until healing is complete.

11. Osteoradionecrosis (ORN) (Figure 6.13)

This is only seen in patients who have had radiotherapy (RT) to the head and neck. To prevent this complication, prior to their RT, any teeth with a poor prognosis should be extracted a few weeks prior to starting RT. Once they have had RT, then these patients should be treated in a hospital setting as they may need pre- and post-dives of hyperbaric oxygen.

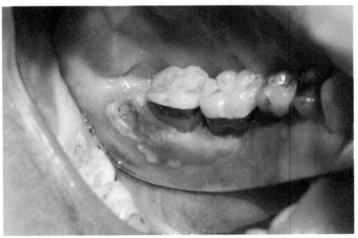

Figure 6.13 ORN of jawbone

12. Medication-related osteonecrosis of the jawbone (MRONJ)

MRONJ refers to an area of exposed or necrotic bone in the maxillofacial region that has not healed within eight weeks, in a patient who has been exposed to an antiresorptive or antiangiogenic medication orally or intravenously and has not had any radiotherapy to the head and neck region.

Patients may experience pain, discomfort, mobile teeth, exposure of dead bone or altered sensation. They may develop secondary infections in these areas. Like ORN, prevention is vital, and patients should be dentally fit prior to commencing therapy. The risk of the patient should be judged, commonly by whether it is oral or IV therapy.

There is no cure for MRONJ, and you are relying on the patient's body to heal up. This is a significant risk that patients must be warned of prior to an extraction.

Any patient with a past medical history of osteoporosis or cancer should be specifically asked about bisphosphonate intake as they may not think it's important to volunteer the information. This has happened recently in a patient who was referred to me for a non-healing post-extraction area (Figure 6.14). This patient has admitted to having IV Fosamax in the past. However, she did not volunteer the information to her dentist prior to extraction.

Ideally, extractions should be avoided at all costs. If you decide to extract the tooth then this is the protocol I follow. I give the patient a Corsodyl rinse for 1 minute pre-op (provided that they are not allergic to it), and then perform the extraction as gently as possible (avoiding disturbance to the periosteum). This is followed by copious saline irrigation to the socket, and I aim to achieve primary closure to preserve the clot and reduce the chance of infection. I also give the patient antibiotics for a week. More importantly, I make sure I review the patient in 8 weeks before they are discharged to their referring dentist.

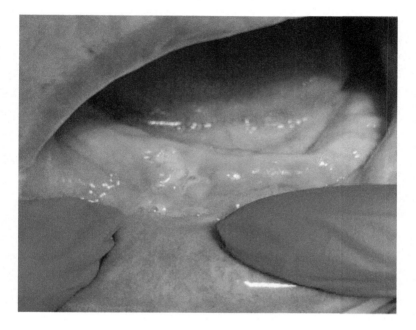

Figure 6.14 MRONJ post lower dental clearance

13. Transmissible viral disease eg, hepatitis, infective endocarditis, Covid-19 or HIV

I can safely say I have seen most of the above complications over the years. Either I have caused them, seen them happen, or had them referred to me for management. I can guarantee that you too will see them, so you had better be prepared to deal with them. I will give you tricks that hopefully will prevent, or make them less likely, for you as a general dentist working in a dental practice, to cause these complications. Only if you pay attention though.

7 The tooth extraction process (how I do it)

Despite the best risk assessment and planning, about 10% of planned forceps extractions become complicated and require some form of surgical approach. That's why you and your team should always be prepared.

Surgical extraction should not be reserved for the most extreme cases. When used appropriately it can be more conservative and cause less morbidity and tissue damage than a forceps extraction, especially when too much force must be applied to extract the tooth which may cause bone and possibly root fracture.

Once again I repeat the consenting process making sure I explain the pros and cons. I clarify what can go wrong during the extraction, and clarify potential post-extraction side effects. When we all know which tooth is to be extracted, and the tooth is perfectly anaesthetised, I almost always start by using a small to medium-sized sharp straight luxator to separate the gum from the tooth, break the periodontal ligament, and gently enlarge the space between the tooth roots and the bone. This enables me to have a feel of the tooth too (how solid it is). Make sure you use the luxator safely (use a finger rest) and never lean on adjacent teeth. Luxators are sharp instruments and the utmost care should be taken when using them to avoid damage to soft tissues.

I then pick up the correct extraction forceps for the tooth to be extracted.

The forceps should be adequately seated and adapted for a successful extraction. They should be placed as apically as possible and reseated periodically during the extraction. The beaks of the forceps should be shaped to adapt to the root of the tooth (Figure 7.1). If they don't, different forceps should be used. The beaks of the forceps should be held parallel to the long axis of the tooth so that the forces generated are delivered along the tooth's long axis. This provides maximal effectiveness in expanding the bone.

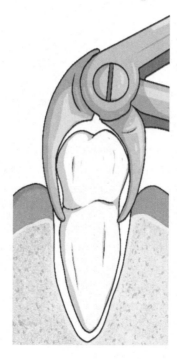

Figure 7.1 Correct grip of forceps on root

I make sure I have a mechanical advantage ie, my arm is extended, and I am above the tooth to be extracted with my legs apart (for upper teeth should be shoulder level and for lower teeth elbow level) (Figure 7.2). I make sure I have enough lighting and magnification, and my trained nurse is ready with the powerful surgical suction (not the wide pore high vacuum one).

You do not have to be strong if you correctly apply the above. It is not about the strength but the technique. The use of excessive force should be avoided, and every effort should be made to develop "feeling" through the forceps. This enables you to recognise resistance to excursions in certain directions and to exploit other movements which the tooth will follow more easily. Therefore always aim to extract along the line of least resistance (listen to the tooth).

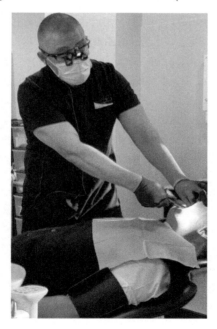

Figure 7.2 Arm straight, legs apart

It is also important that you keep reassuring the patient throughout the procedure and always look and sound confident even if you are running into difficulties. If you lose patient trust, then the whole procedure becomes more difficult and takes even more time.

Simple extraction should usually not take more than 5-10 minutes if risk assessment was carried out properly. If you are taking longer, then you must change your tactic and ask yourself why. If you keep doing the same thing you will not make progress and you will lose the battle and the patient (and possibly his family and friends too). Doing the same thing will achieve the same result.

If the tooth breaks during the extraction, make sure you find and remove the broken fragments from the patient's mouth (risk of inhalation and swallowing). Take a good view of what is left and do a risk assessment (go back to the drawing board). Take a deep breath and ask yourself, do I need to remove the remaining tooth or root or is it OK to leave it alone? If you decide to remove, then it is better to take a radiograph if you have not already done so, to check for root anatomy, bone quality etc. If you decide to leave, then there is no need for a radiograph, just document and inform the patient and offer them a review appointment.

The traditional teaching of how to deal with broken roots during extraction is as follows. Take a radiograph to check the size of the broken roots. If the root tip is more than 5mm then you should remove, and if smaller then leave. Prescribe antibiotics and bring the patient in for a review in a few weeks. This does not make any sense and is unnecessary.

It saves the patient from going through the pain and suffering and avoids the potential risk of damage to important structures like the mental nerve which, if it happens, can't be justified.

Whenever you are doing anything in a patient's mouth, always ask the patient to breathe through their nose. This simple manoeuvre will ensure that it is less likely for them to inhale a broken fragment or even a small instrument.

Do everything you can to avoid fracturing the alveolar plates (mainly labial/buccal) especially if you are planning to place an implant immediately or in the near future. One way to do this is to surgically section the tooth and roots to allow easy and gentle removal of the tooth. Also, avoid buccolingual movement and apply more rotation. I always rotate and figure of eight any tooth without exception.

I have broken many teeth and left many roots of different sizes over the years with minimal or no consequence to the patients.

Sometimes leaving roots behind is advantageous as it means the bone will still be available for future implants if needed (the patient and the implant dentist will thank you for it). When you break a root, ask yourself why you need to take it out rather than leave it behind.

Once the tooth/root is loose, then I grab the correct extraction forceps, apply it to the tooth making sure that the beaks are engaging the crown correctly but holding the root (not the crown). I then make sure I keep the grip on the root by performing slow, steady movements in all directions but maintaining apical pressure all the time. I always stand on the side of the tooth to be extracted except in case of upper left quadrant teeth where I stand at the front right of the patient. This applies to all teeth. However, for upper wisdom teeth I ask the patient to close their mouth and move their mandible towards the side of extraction. This is to stop the coronoid process from impacting against the tooth and preventing its safe delivery. Remember: the only tools you need for upper wisdom teeth are a Warwick James elevator and bayonet forceps. Never use Cryer's, Winter's or large Coupland.

Once the extraction is complete, I irrigate the socket with saline, making sure no fragments are left behind, then I ask the patient to bite on a damp gauze for three to five minutes. I make sure I take the gauze out before the patient leaves the dental chair and make sure haemostasis is achieved.

Either myself or my trained assistant then provides the patient with clear verbal as well as written post-extraction care instructions, including an out of hours telephone number, followed by a care call the day after (first class customer service).

When it comes to the order of teeth extraction, there is no specific order. However, to prevent blood from the sockets of extracted teeth obscuring the field of operation it is usual to remove the lower teeth before the uppers, and posterior teeth before anterior. Always start by extracting the most painful tooth when undertaking multiple extractions just in case you run into complications either surgical or technical, then at least you have relieved the patient of pain.

The canine tends to be the most difficult tooth to extract due to its long conical root usually with a very thin labial plate, therefore this should be extracted last. Extractions of the teeth on either side of the canine weaken its bony housing, potentially making the canine easier to extract.

8 How to prevent extraction complications

Don't do it (only joking). Time spent assessing the problem pre-operatively is never wasted, hence the old saying in carpentry "measure twice and cut once".

The first extraction is always daunting and scary. I still remember my first ever extraction when I was in my third-year dental school (first clinical year) back in my home country Libya. Although it was for LL2, grade two mobile, I was nervous and my hands were shaking. So, make sure to have someone with good clinical experience who is happy to assist and support you should you run into difficulties in your first few extraction cases. Always start with simple ones to build confidence and gain experience.

A. Identify the risks (risk assessment).

B. Investigate to quantify the risks. Take the necessary radiographs or scans if needed to plan and communicate with the patient.

C. Update the PMH. It is very important that a full up to date PMH is taken as it affects patient management (more later).

D. Communicate effectively (with the patient, team, referring clinicians and GP or hospital consultant). The most common cause of complaints and litigations is bad communication.

With proper risk assessment, unexpected complications should not really happen if you follow my recommendations below:

1. Do a thorough risk assessment.

2. Know your patient well (talk to them, build a rapport and in a way become their trusted friend).

3. Be psychologically prepared (mindset). Say to yourself I can do it!

4. Make sure you have the time, a trained nurse, and all the necessary tools and equipment required.

5. Re-consent and double check the tooth to be extracted (remember consent is a continuous process).

6. Achieve profound local anaesthesia. If you can't achieve proper anaesthesia, then you will lose the patient and probably his/her family and friends.

7. Decide if this is a simple or surgical extraction. Always prepare a surgical tray even for a simple extraction. Be prepared.

8. Never let the patient leave until haemostasis is achieved. Do not send them home with a gauze in their mouth.

9. Use the correct elevator/luxator and forceps.

10. Holding the tooth with the correct extraction forceps perform slow, steady movements in all directions, always maintaining APICAL pressure. If you rush, then you may simply convert a simple extraction to a nightmare one.

11. Always be on top of the tooth (correct position). I

always stand on the side of the tooth to be extracted except for the upper left quadrant where I stand on the front right of the patient.

12. Never ask the patient to blow their nose (Valsalva) after extraction of upper posterior teeth. If you cause OAC that is large enough to warrant immediate repair, then you will see it (a hole in the sinus and air bubbles).

13. Spend some time with a specialist surgeon and learn from them. Perform a few extractions under their supervision and mentoring, and get a few cases under your belt.

14. Know your head and neck anatomy inside out especially the 5th and 7th cranial nerves.

15. Practice extraction, raising and suturing flaps on animals or proper rubber models.

16. Do not be scared, especially of governing bodies, if you treat the patient like you would treat your daughter or mother. If you practice defensive dentistry, then you will never make progress or build a prosperous dental practice.

17. You do not have to follow the crowd. Remember, guidelines are ONLY for guidance!

18. Always keep an open mind when you learn from experienced clinicians because they are simply passing their vast experience to you, sometimes for free!

19. There is no excuse for not learning something new every day.

20. Always work in a team and not alone. This way you and your patient will always feel supported.

9 Local anaesthesia secrets

A sound knowledge of anatomy is paramount. All teeth except the lower molars can be extracted with LA infiltration ie, adjacent to the root apex of the tooth to be extracted especially using 4% Articaine with 1:100:000 adrenaline. Although some clinicians advocate the use of infiltration anaesthesia for the extraction of lower molars, in my hands it does not work! (For some reason, it works for implant placement but not for extraction). Keep a mental image of the diagram overleaf (Figure 9.1) to orientate you when giving LA injections for the lower jaw.

Only when you have the knowledge will you have the confidence, and if the patient feels that then you are already a winner. This is most important if the patient is nervous or has had failed anaesthesia before with another dentist. Tell the patient that you use a different technique and stronger anaesthetic so that they will be less nervous and forget about their previous experience. I do not believe in a maximum dose, as in reality there is hardly any situation where you will be injecting more than eight to ten cartridges which should be very safe. In fact, I have never seen any complications related to using too many local anaesthetic cartridges although I quite often use more than 10 (for example for upper and lower clearance or full mouth implants).

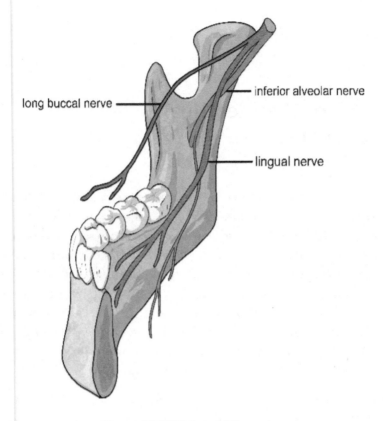

long buccal nerve

inferior alveolar nerve

lingual nerve

Figure 9.1 IDN, L and LB nerves

The anaesthetic agent and total dose administered should be customised to reflect the nature of the procedure and the physical status of the patient. Consideration of patient health status, age, and body weight are more realistic parameters for dose determination than maximum amounts recommended by the manufacturer. The maximum doses are based on the average healthy adult and are not realistic for children, the elderly, or the debilitated patient.

The most common cause of failed LA in my experience is simply not giving enough in the right place. I know some colleagues I have worked with advocate giving only one or two cartridges (of 1.8 ml) for IDN block, lingual and long buccal. However, this is usually not enough, especially for IDN block, due to anatomical difficulties and variations and sometimes difficulty injecting next to the nerve. If adequate anaesthesia is not achieved and the extraction is attempted and the patient feels pain, then the patient may lose confidence. No matter how many more cartridges you give you may still lose, especially if you start poking the gum with a sharp probe and asking the patient whether they can feel anything sharp or not. This habit, which is usually taught at dental schools, is bad and should be abandoned.

Other possible causes include inaccurate placement of the anaesthetic solution and not waiting long enough (rare with the modern solutions), or inappropriate anaesthetic for the planned procedure (eg, infiltration for removal of lower molar).

I have never failed to achieve adequate anaesthesia for extraction of any tooth including lower molars. This is probably because of the following technique:

My technique and secret of success is simple. For lower molar extraction, I use two different LAs and I usually start with 4% Articaine with 1:100:000 adrenaline, and finish off with Articaine in addition to 2% Xylocaine with 1:80:000 adrenaline. For an IDN block I use what I call "the Dalghous double block technique" (DDBT) (Figure 9.3) where I use two cartridges (2 IDN blocks one above the other) and another cartridge for local infiltration all around the tooth to be extracted (lingual, buccal, mesial and distal). Using this technique will ensure:

A. Enough LA is given around the ID nerve before it enters the mandibular canal.

B. Synergism (two different agents potentiate the action of each other).

C. High deposition of LA with different anaesthetic for the second IDN block.

This is a simple technique that requires a slight alteration to the standard mandibular block approach and as such is very easy to employ for increasing success in obtaining mandibular anaesthesia.

The advantages of this approach are its ease of use and the deposition of local anaesthetic higher in the pterygomandibular space allowing for better effectiveness of the local anaesthetic.

1. This technique uses all the same landmarks as a standard IDN block including the coronoid notch, the contralateral premolars and pterygomandibular raphe. In addition, palpate the mandibular notch intraorally to determine the maximum height of injection.

2. Like the standard IDN block (Figure 9.2), use the contralateral premolars to determine the angle of insertion of the needle. Instead of injecting local anaesthetic solution at the level of the coronoid notch, which is approximately 1.0 centimetre above the mandibular occlusal plane (bisecting fingernail), insert the needle so that it contacts the medial aspect of the ramus just below the mandibular notch, a point that is 2.0 centimetres above the mandibular occlusal plane (top edge of your finger) (Figure 9.3). There should be minimal resistance to the injection of local anaesthetic as one is injecting into the potential space of the medial aspect of the mandibular ramus.

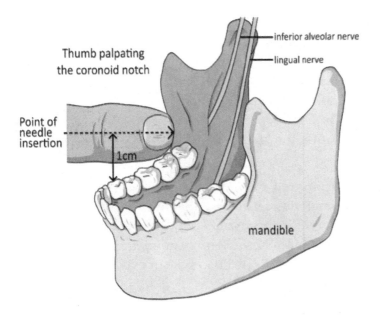

Figure 9.2 Standard technique for IDN block

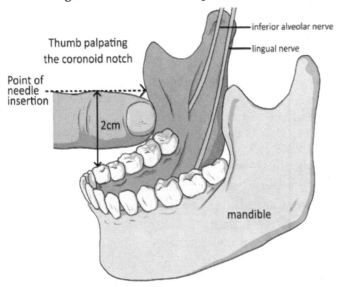

Figure 9.3 "the Dalghous DIDB technique"

After I give the above, I wait for two minutes then I put my right hand on my patient's shoulder, apply pressure and say to the patient, "It is normal to feel pressure like this as we push teeth out, but you should not feel anything sharp. If you do, raise your hand and I will stop immediately". I do this rather than test with a sharp probe and keep asking the patient if they felt it. I find this the key to success.

Of course, I infiltrate all around the tooth, especially lingually, to make sure I have covered all bases. There is a very small theoretical risk that multiple IDN blocks may cause nerve paraesthesia, but the benefit of achieving adequate anaesthesia and completing the proposed treatment will prevent a bad patient experience and loss of confidence in dentistry.

In the case of double block injections, it is easier to palpate bony landmarks at the second attempt as the needle can be manoeuvred in the tissues painlessly. Sometimes it is almost impossible to palpate the lingula which indicates the point of entry of the ID nerve into the mandibular canal or even feel the external oblique ridge which makes the technique difficult, so the above technique helps to achieve anaesthesia even in these situations.

I am also very generous with the amount of anaesthetic I inject. This allows room for inaccurate localisation of the nerve as the liquid spreads and reaches the nerve before it enters the mandibular canal. This is what I teach in my courses whether practical, theoretical or clinical. I only preach what I practice and only teach what I practice routinely. In my practice, there is no maximum dose of anaesthesia in the generally fit and well patient. The idea is that you need to give as much as needed to achieve profound anaesthesia, provided you follow the advice I gave earlier (two different LA, one higher than the other) for an IDN block. However, if you fail to achieve anaesthesia after 4 cartridges then maybe it is a good idea to ask for help from a more experienced colleague.

The other myth in oral surgery is not to give bilateral IDB as it may cause difficulty in breathing! This is not true, and again this is something I do quite often when needed (eg, for the extraction of bilateral wisdom teeth or multiple extractions with or without intravenous sedation).

10 Oral surgery risk assessment

Risk assessment in oral surgery begins with the golden rule. Treat patients the way you would want to be treated yourself, or the way you would want your daughter or mother to be treated.

We all want to receive the highest quality of care in oral surgery. We want our dentists and oral surgeons to listen to our complaints, symptoms and concerns. We want them to evaluate us appropriately through a complete and thorough examination and appropriate diagnostic tests, obtain outside specialist referral when appropriate, consider treatment options, and then discuss those options with us objectively so that we can choose our course of treatment. We want to understand the risks, benefits, and possible complications of our treatment options, including no treatment. We want the process to be legibly documented in our dental records so that it can be reviewed to possibly help with additional challenges that we might face.

How can we minimise the risk associated with any surgical procedure? A quote of the late poet Emily Dickinson put it best when she said, "If you take care of the small things, the big things take care of themselves." An appropriate pre-operative patient assessment is a critical component of surgical success.

Complex oral surgery procedures are occurring more commonly in primary care, performed by both specialist oral surgeons and non-specialists/dentists with a special interest in oral surgery, and by experienced general dentists. This is to reduce the patient load on hospitals, and is due to the increase in the number of private dental practices and the need to retain patients in the practice.

Dentists in the UK are working in an increasingly litigious environment which is often at the forefront of a dentist's mind, and the prevention of complaints and claims of negligence is paramount in maintaining the high standard and confidence in dentistry. Dentists need to be aware of the risks associated with oral surgery procedures and must be able to assess and design a treatment plan that is safe and effective.

It is paramount that as dentists we are aware of our scope of practice and can fully inform patients of the risks and benefits of treatment during the consent process. Dentists must know their limits and when to refer patients on to a colleague with more surgical experience, a specialist or hospital.

Oral surgery is often an unpleasant experience for patients and, if managed inadequately, can be a cause for complaint or a claim of negligence. A dentist can reduce their risk of complaints, claims or even regulatory body investigations, not by refusing to treat the patient but by simply following some straightforward risk assessment. An honest reflection by the practitioner on their competence to carry out a procedure, considering their skills, the equipment and support available, will result in fewer medico-legal cases.

Extraction of teeth is the bread and butter for general dentists and, provided a proper risk assessment of each case is done, there is no excuse in my opinion for any dentist to refer simple and moderately difficult extractions in patients with no medical contraindications to a specialist or hospital. Fear of litigation or complaint is not an excuse. Imagine saying to a family member, "I need to refer you to a hospital which is many miles away. I know you have no private transport, and you may need two to three buses to get there only to be told your case is not urgent. You will have to wait a few months if not years to be seen for treatment." In addition, if you run your private practice then it may mean you lose the income of that patient and probably his family and friends. Moreover, the extraction of teeth may be part of extensive and expensive restorative treatment for that patient. If you do not have the skills and competence to do the simple extraction, then you may not only lose money but more importantly not be able to help the patient achieve their perfect smile, and improve their oral health and wellbeing. Time taken to get to know the patient and doing a risk assessment is never wasted.

I encourage every newly qualified dentist to spend some time either in a hospital or in a primary care setting shadowing and learning from a specialist surgeon, or even a dentist with experience in oral surgery, to learn and increase their confidence. Believe me, oral surgery skills are easy if you learn from the right person and practice as many cases as possible under their supervision (on animal models and of course real patients).

Once you master the skills then there will be a very limited number of cases that need hospital, or specialist care.

I am not by any means underestimating or oversimplifying teeth extraction, but what I am saying is it is a skill that is very simple to learn and enjoy if you work in the right environment. I am very lucky to work within a team where each team member knows that they are supported all the time by each other. We discuss cases and formulate plans together, and when patients see that they gain more confidence and feel they are in safe hands and are being well looked after. We have a culture of openness and respect for each other. No one knows it all.

Unfortunately, most if not all newly qualified dentists aspire to be cosmetic dentists and they forget about not only oral surgery and oral medicine skills but also general dentistry, caries removal, and simple restorations. Some of them don't even know their head and neck anatomy or even how to do a proper full head and neck examination. They only look at teeth in isolation, and decide to make the shape and colour better by means of veneers, crowns, composite bonding and teeth whitening. What about the soft tissue and examination of at least high risk areas especially in patients who smoke and drink alcohol? All dentists should think like a physician and have the skills of an excellent surgeon.

All you need to do is know your anatomy and physiology (the normal), and pathology (the abnormal) to be able to diagnose the problem (the disease) and formulate a proper management plan.

Know what investigations are required to reach a diagnosis and then formulate a treatment plan. Discuss the plan and options with the patient in an honest and open way, including options that may be beyond your remit.

Do a risk assessment based on your assessment, chatting with the patient etc.

Risk assessment is a big topic and in my opinion is the most important topic.

Risk assessment starts from first patient contact, which is usually either via the practice website, social media or a phone call to the front of house team. At this first phone call, very valuable information can be gathered from listening to the patient and their reasons for contacting the practice and making notes that can be accessed by the clinician.

The patient's story and the reason for their call may give you information about the experience the patient has had, their expectations, and whether they are nervous etc. All the information should be recorded in the patient notes and profile so the dentist will have an idea about the patient before face-to-face consultation and examination takes place.

When I first meet a patient, I greet them with a big smile and shake their hand. I introduce myself, and then we sit on a sofa in a non-clinical area making sure that I am sitting on the same side as they are. I have a relaxed chat with them, establish a rapport, and listen to their concerns. I show empathy and reiterate what they have discussed with me to assure them that I fully understand their concerns. Then we go to the surgery and I complete a full and thorough head and neck examination. I always start by examining extraorally (lymph nodes, V and IIV cranial nerves, symmetry etc) then intraorally (floor of mouth, cheeks, lips, oropharynx etc).

Failure to do a proper risk assessment may turn a relatively simple extraction into a complicated problem of management. It can even lead to the inability to complete the procedure, and possible litigation. Risk assessment can be divided into:

A. Patient factors

B. Clinical factors

C. Radiographic findings

D. Operator and team-related factors

A. Patient factors

Assessment starts from the phone call taken by the reception team (see above). The first contact with the patient is very important. Patient anxiety, age, gender, build, race (eg Afro Caribbean) (Figure 10.1), disability (wheelchair user, kyphosis or severe ankylosing spondylitis), profession and habits (bruxism), history of difficult extraction, isolated teeth (hypercementosis) are all very important factors in assessing the difficulty of extraction. For example, in old age the roots of the teeth are brittle and the bone is more sclerosed, the so-called 'glass in concrete syndrome'.

In my practice, the way I assess the patient is as follows. As soon as I see the patient, especially if they were referred to me, I can tell straight away, before I even ask the patient to open their mouth, whether the extraction is more likely to be easy or difficult. If the patient is very nervous, well built (rugby player or body builder), or an Afro Caribbean old male, then I know to get the surgical kit and the drill out.

Then after taking a full PMH and dental history, including the reason for attendance, I examine them. I assess their mouth opening (microstomia, trismus), masticatory muscles' tone, accessibility, position and condition of the tooth or root to be extracted, and then I take a radiograph or CBCT (if indicated). Sometimes you can't even palpate the external oblique ridge or visualise the pterygomandibular space, large strong tongue, which make it hard to achieve an IDN block.

The following factors may indicate a challenging or difficult extraction even for the experienced surgeon:

1. isolated, decayed, heavily restored or root treated tooth at the back of the mouth, surrounded by thick alveolar bone or near bony exostosisor tori (Figure 10.2),

2. a large tongue,

3. a severe gag reflex,

4. a nervous patient due to a previous bad experience and history of failed LA,

5. the end of the day on Friday.

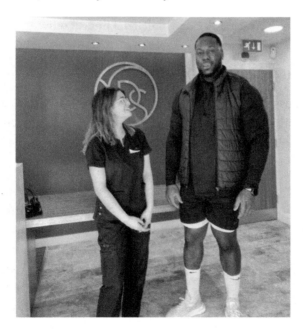

Figure 10.1 Sex, age and ethnicity and build factors

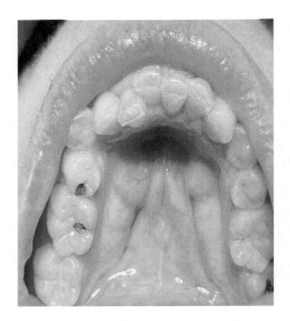

Figure 10.2 Large bilateral lingual tori

B. Clinical factors

1. Access (can the patient get into the chair, degree of mouth opening, size of tongue, size of masseter muscles, gag reflex, skeletal relationship).

2. Related to the tooth to be extracted: location in the mouth (the more posterior the harder), degree of eruption or impaction (the deeper the impaction the harder), extent of decay (how much sound tooth structure is left), crowding (more common in lower anteriors and premolars), risk of damage to teeth and difficult to mobilise crowded teeth, thickness of cortical plates of the jaw, tori (making bone expansion during extraction harder with more risk of fracture of bone and tooth), status of adjacent teeth, oral hygiene (poor

oral hygiene means bleeding gums and increased risk of infection), related structures like nerves and sinus.

3. The more complex the medical history, the more complicated is the management.

4. Assessment of patient cooperation: LA only? Sedation? GA?

C. Radiographic factors

It is not necessary to take a radiograph prior to teeth extraction but it is desirable in the following circumstances:

A. History of difficult extraction. Shed some light on the reasons for the difficulty, which could be the shape, number of roots or hypercementosis.

B. Abnormal resistance to extraction. Excessive force can cause unnecessary damage. It may convert a simple extraction to a difficult surgical one, or may cause extensive dentoalveolar fracture or even mandibular fracture. Find out the reason and deal with it. Don't just carry on doing the same thing. If you can't mobilise the tooth after a few minutes, then find out why.

C. All impacted teeth. How deep? Anatomical structures? Ankyloses?

D. Pathology preventing eruption.

E. Number, shape and size of roots. Again, decide if simple or surgical extraction is needed.

F. Degree of impaction. The deeper the impaction the harder is the surgical extraction.

G. Proximity to anatomical structures (sinus, nerve

(Figures 10.3 and 10.4), etc). Plan for safe extractions to avoid OAC or nerve damage.

H. Ankylosis or hypercementosis

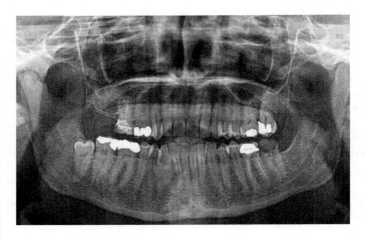

Figure 10.3 Close proximity of LR8 to IDN canal

D. Operator and team-related factors

1. Experience of operator and assistants. More experienced operators are always more accurate in doing the risk assessment for tooth extraction which is the most important thing. Also an experienced assistant makes it easier for the surgeon to do their job properly by not blocking the surgeon's view of the surgical site, by proper aspiration and retraction of soft tissues. The assistant also knows the plan and what the patient has consented to, and this will ensure the safe treatment of the patient. An experienced nurse is always a step ahead and knows what the surgeon needs next (like an experienced chess player). Therefore, time invested in training your nurse to make your job easier is never wasted.

2. Time of the day (tiredness at the end of a day). If you are tired or not feeling great, then it is better to postpone the surgical extraction to another day as tiredness may negatively affect your judgement and in turn complicate the procedure.

3. Surgical kit. Do you have a surgical kit including surgical drill and burs, sutures etc? Do not attempt the extraction of difficult teeth unless you have the facilities for surgical extraction. It is well worth investing in a good surgical kit and surgical straight handpiece and burs (rose head and straight fissure). There are plenty of options on the market and they do not have to be expensive.

Algorithm for risk assessment:

This can be divided into 4 main factors:

A. patient factors

B. clinical factors

C. radiological factors

D. operator factors

A. patient factors

		Score
Age:	Below 40 years	0
	Above 40 years	1
Gender:	Female	0
	Male	1
Ethnicity:	Other	0
	Afro Caribbean	1
Build:	Average and Thin	0
	Tall and Heavy	1
H/O difficult extractions:		
	No	0
	Yes	1
Anxiety:	No	0
	Yes	1
ASA:	I & II	0
	III & IV1	

B. clinical factors

		Score
Tooth to be extracted:	Sound and fully erupted	0
	Fully erupted and carious	1
	Impacted	1
	Malpositioned	1
Site in the mouth:	Front	0
	Posterior	1
Mouth opening:	Normal	0
	Restricted	1
Local anatomy:	Normal	0
	Tori and exostosis	1

C. radiological factors

		Score
Roots:	Single	0
	Multiple	1
Ankylosed:	No	0
	Yes	1
Close to IDN/sinus	No	0
	Yes	1

D. operator factors

		Score
Number of teeth extracted by the dentist:	More than 200	0
	Less than 200	1
Time of day:	Early morning midweek	0
	Late afternoon on a Friday	1

A score of 0 is more likely to be simple extraction

A score of 1-9 is more likely to be surgical extraction

A score of 10 and above may need a specialist or hospital referral

How to risk assess for OAC:

Always take an X-ray for any tooth posterior to the canine. OAC is extremely common after extraction, but we never check for it as it spontaneously heals without problems.

Be aware of enlarged sinus, divergent roots, long standing molar, thick buccal plate (Afro Caribbean), hypercementosis, or heavily restored teeth. Avoid apical pressure with luxators as this may push the root into the sinus. Have a low threshold for surgical extraction when you break roots or when there is no tooth movement with reasonable force, designing the flap for OAC closure if needed. Do not try to retrieve the broken roots blindly even if they are loose. I have seen it enough times where the dentist tries to retrieve a root which seems to be loose and easy to retrieve only to see it disappear into the breached sinus. This is most common when the roots are chronically infected, and the sinus lining is thin and friable. Raise a three-sided full thickness mucoperiosteal flap and release the periosteum so it is easy to advance and close if OAC is created.

11 Management of impacted wisdom teeth

The extraction of symptomatic wisdom teeth remains one of the most performed procedures in primary and secondary care settings.

Nevertheless, it is an operation with a relatively high complication rate which increases among older patients and occasionally leads to claims for negligence. This complication rate can be significantly reduced by early assessment and removal of wisdom teeth.

The most impacted teeth are upper and lower wisdom teeth followed by maxillary canines and lower premolars. NICE guidance has been developed and was aimed to decrease the overall number of wisdom teeth removals. However, there is mounting evidence that wisdom teeth surgery is merely being delayed, bringing with it a variety of problems for the patients. These range from increased prevalence of caries (Figure 11.1) and periodontal disease of the second molar and third molars as well as increased difficulty of surgery, to decreased quality of life and a potentially life-threatening deep space abscess formation following wisdom teeth infection. Considering this and the limited amount of high-quality evidence available, it is this author's opinion that patients should have more autonomy and be offered prophylactic wisdom teeth removal privately, and on the NHS, following consolidation of the associated risks and benefits of the treatment, thorough clinical and radiographic examination, and on a case-by-case basis considering relevant medical history.

It is important to remember that while NICE advises against the extraction of pathology-free impacted wisdom teeth in their guidance, it is merely that – guidance; a tool to aid clinical decision-making.

Risk assessment should be performed, and informed consent should be obtained, rather than sticking to the guidelines categorically. Remember they are only guidelines.

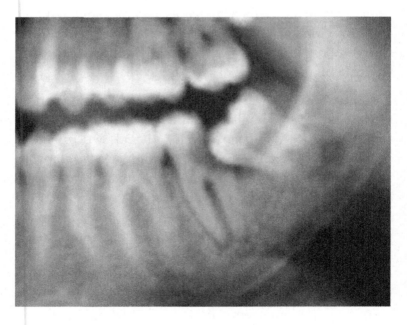

Figure 11.1 Partially erupted LL8 causing decay to LL7

A lengthy discussion, a thorough examination and investigations which may include DMFT (decayed, missing and filled permanent teeth) rate, degree of periodontal disease, OPT or CBCT should be undertaken as part of the assessment and the decision should be made accordingly. Following the guidelines blindly contributes to the large number of older patients needing removal not only of their impacted, now difficult to remove, wisdom teeth but also the adjacent symptomatic unrestorable second molars.

I see this in my clinical practice every day and I consider this as supervised neglect. Complications of wisdom teeth increase in older people due to sclerosis of the bone, and ankylosis of teeth and increased morbidity due to the increased incidence of medical conditions and medications.

In my opinion, wisdom teeth should be removed unless there is a specific contraindication. For example, radiographic evidence of very close proximity of the impacted wisdom tooth to the inferior dental nerve (IDN). This is part of preventive dentistry to prevent disease and complications. There should be a place for removing lower wisdom teeth prophylactically at a younger age where patients are usually healthier with more flexible bone, and roots not fully formed, which makes the procedure easier. In older age, bone becomes more rigid and becomes less forgiving of the forces required to remove these teeth. This means more bone removal and more trauma to the tissue and possibly more complications. In my opinion, this is mainly because dentists are not competent and confident in taking out wisdom teeth, or they simply follow the guidelines categorically. However, prophylactic removal of wisdom teeth should not be performed if the risks outweigh the benefits.

We should be asking ourselves "Why leave them in?" rather than "Why take them out?". If you can't decide, or you don't have the time or the expertise to have a lengthy chat with the patient, then it's better to at least refer them to a specialist to have that chat. Don't just use the guidelines as an excuse to deny the patient the correct treatment which might improve the patient's quality of life and save them potential complications in the future. All GDPs should be able to assess and evaluate wisdom teeth to decide whether extraction is indicated, and whether they can do it in surgery or should refer to a specialist.

Indications for extraction of wisdom teeth

These include, but are not limited to, the following:

1. Recurrent pericoronitis. This is the most common cause for the removal of impacted or partially erupted lower wisdom teeth. It is the infection of the soft tissue flap around the crown of a partially erupted tooth (Figure 11.2). Acute pericoronitis can be serious and life threatening if it spreads to facial and neck spaces. Trauma from a buccally erupting upper wisdom tooth can worsen infection.

2. Periodontal disease.

3. Pathology (cyst) (Figure 11.3).

4. Unrestorable caries of the wisdom tooth or the adjacent tooth (Figure 11.4).

5. Resorption of adjacent tooth roots.

6. Orthognathic surgery.

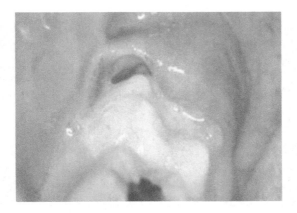

Figure 11.2 Acute pericoronitis associated with partially erupted LR8

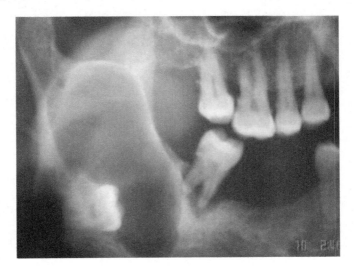

Figure 11.3 Cystic lesion associated with impacted LR8

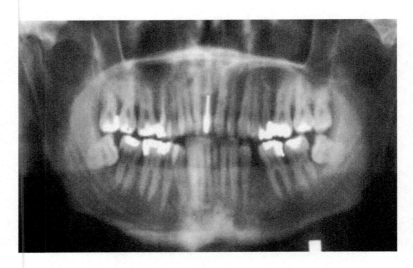

Figure 11.4 Decay LR7 and LL7

12 Surgical removal of lower wisdom teeth (how I do it)

1. Local anaesthesia for IDN, L and LB as described above.

2. Flap: I always use a two-sided flap (Figure 12.1). I stand on the side of the tooth to be removed, ask the patient to open wide to gain access, and stretch the tissue for an easy cut (cutting through a fully inflated balloon is easier than a half inflated one). I cut a full thickness mucoperiosteal flap using a 15c blade, starting from the distobuccal cusp of the lower 7 posteriorly but buccally along the external oblique ridge (remember more buccal than you think). If you are not on bone, then DO NOT CUT. Then I cut a relieving incision between the 8 and the 7 (if I need greater access then I extend it between 7 and 6, (Figure 12.2) including the papilla down towards the mucogingival line. As I cross the mucogingival line I curve it slightly anterior to give me more access. I always make sure I cut towards me for better control of the blade and to ensure I do not slip and cause damage.

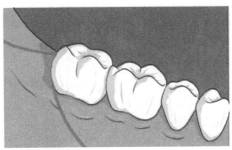

Figure 12.1 2-sided flap for L8 (my standard technique)

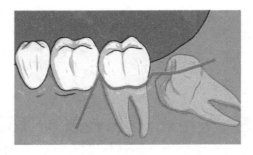

Figure 12.2 Relieving incision extended between 7 & 8 for larger access

I reflect the flap using a blunt elevator and then I place a Lacs retractor. The next step is planning the bone and tooth removal. I use a straight surgical handpiece with copious saline irrigation and a rose head or round bur at 40,000 rpm. I very rarely use fissure bur (sometimes I use it to make a precise cut when dividing the roots that are close to IDN). I drill away as much bone as I need, always bearing in mind that bone is a precious commodity. I also make sure that I am aware as to where the tip of the bur is, as if I go too deep I may cause damage to vital structures like the ID or mental nerve.

I make a buccal gutter and expose the cemento-enamel junction (CEJ) of the tooth, then decide to section the tooth vertically (Figure 12.3) or horizontally.

There is no hard and fast rule when it comes to tooth sectioning - except in the case of distoangular impaction (Figure 12.4). Here, I always section the crown horizontally which makes the tooth not impacted against the ramus of the mandible anymore and also enables me to see the root furcation. I am careful not to section the tooth fully buccolin-gually as there is a risk of going through the lingual cortex and cutting the lingual nerve. Once the tooth is removed, I inspect the socket for debris or extra roots and make sure all is clean. I irrigate with copious amounts of saline including irrigation under the flap. Finally, I suture the socket with resorbable 3/0 or 4/0 sutures and achieve haemostasis.

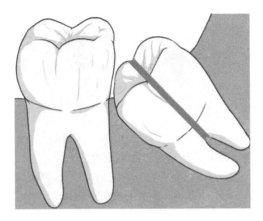

Figure 12.3 Vertical cut through crown LL8

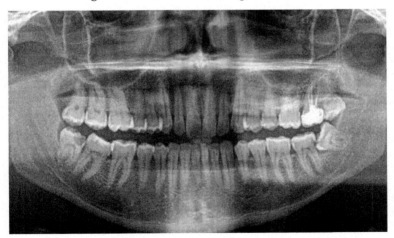

Figure 12.4 Distoangular impacted LR7 and mesioangular LL8

PS Please watch my YouTube video for the procedure (already more than 3 million views): https://youtu.be/ gt7o7Q1bUr8

Coronectomy

The incidence of temporary and permanent inferior dental nerve (IDN) damage following the surgical removal of third molars varies according to author and report, but is in the order of 1–5% for temporary effects and 0–0.9% for permanent deficit. Some authors quote higher figures, with 'high risk' teeth associated with risk as great as 20%.

Coronectomy, defined as "deliberate vital root retention", should be considered in all impacted teeth extractions, especially if there is a clear indication of proximity to the IDN (lower wisdom teeth) or mental nerve (eg, impacted premolars or supernumerary teeth).

Coronectomy is a procedure designed to avoid injury to the IDN by retaining the roots of symptomatic, vital, lower third molar teeth that are close to the inferior dental canal. It is a relatively new technique and is not practiced worldwide. However, in certain cases, if coronectomy is not offered as a treatment option, in my opinion this should be considered medical negligence. It is very important to master coronectomy as it is extremely technique sensitive.

Coronectomy is contraindicated in teeth with active infection, mobile teeth and deep horizontal impaction.

The way I perform a coronectomy is as follows:

I achieve adequate anaesthesia (usually IDN block, buccal and lingual infiltration). I raise a full thickness mucoperiosteal flap as described above then, using a round or rose head surgical bur, I remove bone buccally until I see the CEJ of the 8. I section the crown horizontally 2-3 mm below the CEJ. I make sure that I cut through the crown completely, taking care not to drill the lingual plate and cause damage to the lingual nerve (Figure 12.5). I use very minimum pressure on luxation and elevation of the sectioned crown as this is when it is likely for the roots to become loose, in which case they must be removed too. I then smooth any enamel spurs and reduce the height of the roots a few millimetres below the crest of the alveolar ridge. I do not touch the pulp chamber, and I close the flap with resorbable sutures.

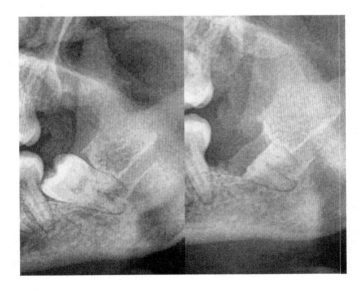

Figure 12.5 Pre and post coronectomy LL8
Picture courtesy of Dr Christine Wanis

13 What should you do when things go wrong?

1. Do not panic!

2. Recognise it and accept it.

3. Be open and honest with your patient.

4. Be objective, factually accurate, but empathetic. Choose your words carefully when explaining to the patient what has happened, and do not cause them to panic. Reassure them that all is under control, because if they panic then that will make it even more stressful for you.

5. Make a prompt and reasonable effort to correct the situation. If you are doing an extraction and the tooth snapped for example, then stop and assess the situation. Have a clear visibility and do a risk assessment (back to the drawing board).

6. Seek senior or expert advice. If you are working in a team with mixed skills and different experience, then go and ask for help. They may give you advice or take over the management of your patient. Once the situation is sorted then make sure you reflect and ask for feedback from the experienced clinician who helped you with the situation.

7. Document the events accurately and honestly.

8. Contact your indemnity for advice. They will always be there for you to give you advice and guidance.

14 Flaps in oral surgery

Flaps in oral surgery are used to allow for complete access and visualisation of the surgical field, to allow for bone removal and tooth sectioning, and to prevent unnecessary damage to soft tissue and bony structures.

All flaps for oral surgery must be mucoperiosteal (full thickness). This flap includes the overlying gingiva, mucosa, submucosa, and underlying periosteum in one piece.

Do not worry too much about the name of the incision, design or shape of the flap. The shape of the incision must be planned with the need of both exposure and closure in mind.

A flap needs to be raised in order to facilitate bone removal and sectioning of the tooth and roots under direct vision to expedite extraction. They should be large enough to permit clear access to the surgical site without stretching and possibly tearing the soft tissues. Ideally the base of the flap should be wider than the free margin to maintain adequate blood supply. Most importantly, when designing a flap make sure you avoid vital structures, especially the mental nerve and lingual nerve. If you need to raise a flap to gain access, visibility, and to make life easy for you, then be generous. A long incision heals as fast as a short incision (healing proceeds across, not along, the incision) so why compromise? If you can see what you are doing, then the rest is easy! It saves you time and energy.

Of course, be aware of the local anatomy, especially nerves. Avoid touching papillae in the aesthetic zone (premolars to premolars) if possible. As a rule, when you hold the blade it should be at 90° to the bone, cutting with the belly. Hold the scalpel handle like a pen. Using a scalpel with a number 15c blade, make sure you cut firmly towards you (this way you have more control as opposed to cutting away from you), down to the bone in a single clean stroke (no see-sawing). The neater the cut the less is the post-operative inflammation and swelling. Be kind to the tissues.

Plan where the incision is going to start and end. When you cut, make sure the tissue is tight for easy incision (remember the inflated balloon analogy). Use plenty of LA containing adrenalin as infiltration for good haemostasis and analgesia.

Although generous in extent, bone removal must be calculated to achieve an end, and never be blindly destructive. The main objectives should be the achievement of access, the establishment of a point of application for an elevator (or forceps), and removal of the obstruction to movement of the tooth or root.

Teach your nurse/assistant how to assist you. Use surgical suction with a fine tip to aspirate blood and fluid efficiently. Teach her not to obstruct your vision while aspirating. Use loupes with adequate magnification and lighting.

Despite the benefits of raising a flap, many dentists will try to avoid doing it, either because of inexperience or a lack of training. But the alternative - for example attempting to remove a broken tooth by persistently digging at it within the socket - can be a nightmare for both dentist and patient. Very often I see patients referred to me for failed extraction who tell me that the dentist tried for more than an hour or two to remove the broken fragment before they gave up.

Most used flaps are one-sided or envelope (Figure 14.1), two (Figure 14.2) or three-sided (Figure 14.3 and 14.4) and semilunar (Figure 14.5) or rectangular (Figure 14.6).

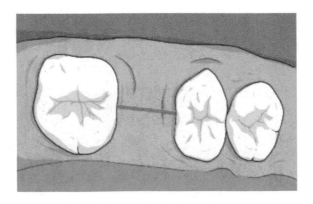

Figure 14.1 Envelope flap

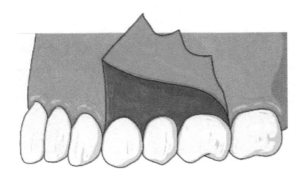

Figure 14.2 Two-sided flap

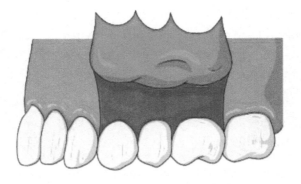

Figure 14.3 Three-sided flap

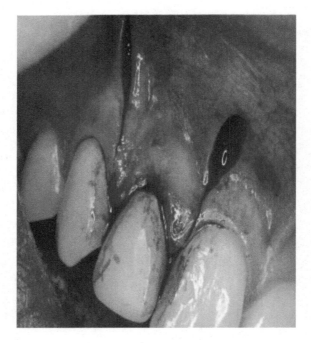

Figure 14.4 Three-sided flap

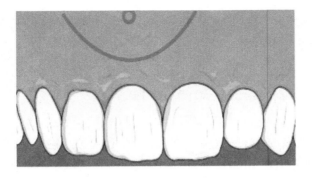

Figure 14.5 Semilunar flap

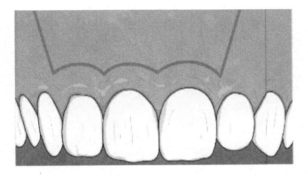

Figure 14.6 Rectangular flap

In most cases I always start with a two-sided flap with one incision along the gingival margin and another, called a relieving incision, angled obliquely across the attached buccal gingiva into the lax vestibular mucosa (crossing the mucogingival junction). This relieving incision should be mesial to the most anterior tooth to allow extension in a distal direction if required. This design gives adequate access for most surgical extractions including wisdom teeth. If greater access is required, then this flap can be easily converted to a three-sided flap by having a second relieving incision at the distal end of the flap. This is mainly used to close OAC/OAF or for peri radicular surgery.

115

My least favourable flap is the semilunar or rectangular, the main indication of which is peri radicular surgery associated with crowned teeth to avoid disturbing the gingival margin. Its disadvantages can be an unsightly scar and inadequate access (Figure 14.7).

When raising a flap, make sure it is easy to accurately suture and put the tissues back where they belong without tension. This can be made easy by including the full thickness of the interdental papilla in the flap (never bisect the papilla) (Figure 14.8).

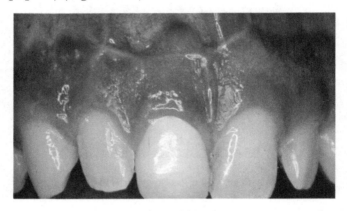

Figure 14.7 Unsightly scarring

Raise the full thickness flap using a periosteal elevator under the anterior edge of the flap where the relieving incision is through the vestibular mucosa, not the attached gingiva (harder). Once you are in the right plane, stay in contact with the bone. Push backwards and the flap should slide easily if it was full thickness. If it does not raise with ease, then you may have to revise your incision and make sure you cut down to the bone with a fresh blade (once it touches bone the blade becomes blunt). When the flap is raised, use a suitable retractor such as a Lacs Minnesota to hold the flap out of the surgical site and retract the lip or cheek at the same time. Avoid repositioning the retractor to minimise trauma to the flap. The minimum the trauma, the smoother is the recovery and the minimum bruising and swelling (the difference between good surgery and a bad one is the way you handle the tissue).

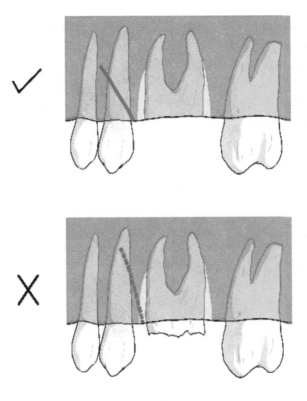

Figure 14.8 Do not bisect papilla

15 Suturing

For suturing oral incisions you need a needle holder, blunt-ended sharp scissors, fine-toothed dissecting forceps (not hospital tweezers), suture materials and skills.

You need a selection of suture material (absorbable and non-absorbable) of different sizes. It is better to use absorbable so that the patient does not have to come back to see you to have the sutures removed, especially if they travel from afar. The most versatile needle is about 19-22mm in length, a curvature of 3/8th of the circumference of a circle, and reverse cutting. I almost always use 4/0 and 3/0 resorbable sutures. Suture size refers to the diameter of the material. The larger the number, the smaller the diameter of the material (eg, 5/0 is smaller than 3/0).

1. The most common suturing techniques I use are interrupted and mattress suture (vertical and horizontal). The best way to learn suturing is to observe an oral surgeon and practice at home on a banana skin, sponge or artificial gum.

2. Insert the needle at a right angle to the tissue about 3mm from the gingival margin (base of papilla) to ensure enough bite of tissue and avoid tearing when tying it up. Also, start from the free edge to the attached

and take one bite at a time.

3. Avoid tight knots as these may restrict the blood supply and delay healing (approximate NOT strangulate).

4. Pass the needle through one side at a time to ensure accuracy, and place the knot to one side of the wound (usually buccally) rather than directly over it.

5. Sutures should be placed 2-3mm apart. In the case of extraction wounds, they should be placed in the interdental papilla, not in the middle of the socket.

6. Although you can hand tie, it is better and easier to tie the knot with a needle holder.

16 Extraction in high risk and medically compromised patients

Due to advances in medical care and health awareness, patients now live much longer as compared to a century ago. It means you are more likely to treat frail old patients who are immunocompromised or on poly pharmacy that may affect the planned treatment. Update the PMH at each visit and make a note of any changes. Ask about any complications from previous extractions. I believe that to be a great surgeon you must be a great physician!

There are no absolute contraindications for extractions, and I have never had to turn any patient away for medical reasons. However, there are precautions and necessary steps that must be taken to ensure safe management of the patient. In addition, communication with the patient's GP, treating consultant, and referring dentist is paramount to ensure a smooth journey with minimum or no complications. This also avoids litigation of negligence and suboptimal patient care.

The only patients in my opinion who need treatment under hospital care are those who have had previous RT to the jaws and are at risk of ORN, patients with coagulation and bleeding problems, and patients who are on a high therapeutic range of warfarin (INR of 4 or above).

Prophylactic extraction of all symptomatic teeth with a poor prognosis should be performed at least a few weeks prior to starting RT or bisphosphonates treatment. If this opportunity is missed, and the patient presents to clinic with acute symptoms, then referral to hospital is indicated. All other patients can be safely treated in a primary care setting with some modifications and adaptations to their management. Sending patients away to hospital without thinking is not a good option especially if you run your own private practice.

17 Orofacial infections and their management in the dental practice

It is not uncommon for patients to attend your practice as an emergency due to acute dentoalveolar infection.

Infections should be treated promptly and aggressively to avoid complications. These complications include spread to potential facial spaces and airway compromise, blindness due to orbital or intracranial spread, loss of bone and teeth, scarring and sinus tract formation, and facial disfigurement.

Orofacial infections can lead to sepsis which can lead to tissue damage, organ failure and death.

The overall principle of surgical intervention is:

1. Identify and eliminate the source of infection.

2. Incise for drainage.

3. Carry out blunt dissection.

4. Copiously irrigate with saline.

5. Maintain drainage for 48-72 hours.

When a patient attends for an appointment with a dental infection, most dentists feel overwhelmed and automatically assume that dealing with the infection is out of their skillset. They subsequently refer the patient to a hospital for specialist care. This simply should not be the case, as most orofacial infections have a simple solution in the form of treatment. In this chapter I have devised a formula to simplify, and help you to understand, the safe and effective management of dental infections in a primary care setting.

Management of any dental abscess is surgical never medical (ie, antibiotics). However, the distinction should be made between a localised abscess and a spreading cellulitis. Do not prescribe antibiotics and hope for the best just because you do not have the skills to appropriately manage the situation. The patient may develop tolerance to antibiotics, or worse still may suffer an anaphylactic reaction and could die. Please think twice before you prescribe them.

Most encountered dental infections are acute dental abscesses or pericoronitis.

Localised signs and symptoms of acute pericoronitis are pain and tenderness of an operculum, with a bad taste from discharging pus. However, there may also be systemic involvement and trismus.

Treatment of acute pericoronitis depends on severity and systemic involvement. It usually presents as pain and tenderness associated with a partially erupted lower wisdom tooth. It is due to the accumulation of plaque and debris under the operculum (Figure 17.1).

Management is simply by reassurance, irrigation with copious saline under the operculum, plus or minus extraction of the upper wisdom tooth if it is causing trauma to the operculum. Also, frequent warm salt mouth rinses and NSAID.

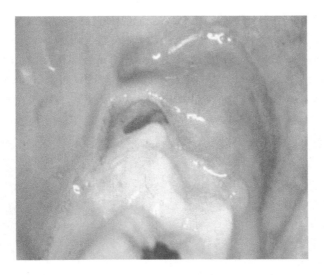

Figure 17.1 Acute pericoronitis associated with partially erupted LR8

If there is systemic involvement, then prescribe antibiotics in the form of amoxicillin 500mg TDS or metronidazole 400mg TDS if the patient has no allergies.

If the tooth is easy to extract, then extraction is the best option. If referral to a specialist or secondary care is indicated based on risk assessment, then the above measures should suffice. The patient should be shown how to irrigate and a monojet syringe should be dispensed.

In my experience, operculectomy does not work. I feel it is a waste of time and money, and is a surgical insult to the patient.

A dry socket is not an infection and should not be treated with antibiotics alone.

The basic principles of management include obtaining drainage (if there is collection) and controlling the spread of infection with antibiotics. Controlling a localised collection with antibiotics alone is inadequate.

The most important clinical decision to be made is whether the swelling represents an abscess (a collection of pus, Figure 17.2) or cellulitis (rapidly spreading infection, Figure 17.3). An abscess demands surgical intervention, whereas cellulitis is best managed medically at least until signs of abscess formation occur.

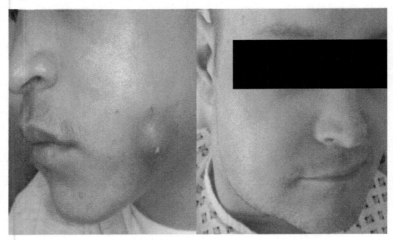

Figure 17.2   **Figure 17.3**

Abscess with draining sinus   **Spreading cellulitis**

Each dental surgery should be equipped with a non-invasive BP measuring machine, pulse oximeter and thermometer.

Antibiotics should not be the treatment of choice for a localised infection and abscess formation. Treatment of a dental abscess is surgical and is by identification and elimination of the cause, and drainage of the abscess. This can be achieved by either drainage through the tooth (if the tooth is a strategic one and needs to be saved), or extraction of the tooth and incision and drainage. Only if there is spreading infection (cellulitis) should antibiotics be used to limit the spread.

Drainage should be correctly performed making sure all loci of infections are broken. A drain may be inserted and secured with sutures for a few days until all the pus is drained (use a corrugated or rubber glove drain). Once you drain the abscess make sure you irrigate with copious amounts of saline (dilution is the solution to pollution). Always make sure you give the patient a contact number and give them a care call the day after to check they are making an adequate recovery.

In patients with a severe orofacial abscess, achieving adequate anaesthesia can be tricky, and a nerve block anaesthesia may be necessary. Avoid injecting into the infected area as theoretically it may facilitate the spread of infection and may not be effective.

Check their vital signs including temperature, pulse, BP, O_2 saturation.

Intraoral:

Do they have free tongue movement? Ask patient to stick their tongue out and check for free movement. Is the tongue elevated? protruded?

Floor of mouth - is it soft or firm and elevated?

Swelling/collection. Any inflammatory oedema or collection, and its origin (teeth, gum)?

Teeth (carious, TTP, mobile)? Usually, infected teeth are easy to remove (Figure 17.4).

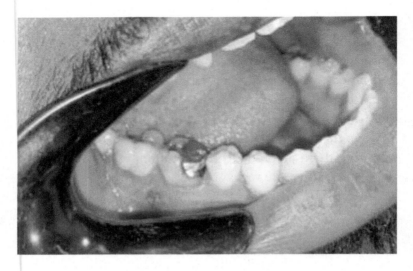

Figure 17.4 Draining sinus related to non-vital LR6

Radiographs/CBCT findings:

PA area?

Deep pocket?

Cortication (chronicity), no cortication (acute infection, Figure 17.5)

Anatomy (roots, nerves, sinus)

If the patient is cooperative and consented for extraction of the offending tooth and drainage of the abscess, then aim to complete today. Extract the tooth, copiously irrigate with saline, and drain the abscess.

There is no need for antibiotics if there is no systemic manifestation of bacteraemia. Advise home rest, fluids and analgesics. Make a follow up call the next day.

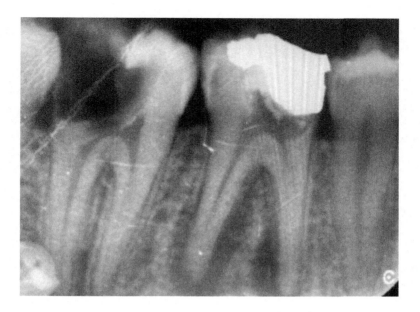

Figure 17.5 Acute PA abscess LR6 - note absence of cortication

Indications for referral of a patient with dentofacial infection to hospital include:

1. Signs of severity

- Fever

- Dehydration

- Rapid increase of swelling

- Trismus

- Elevation of tongue

- Swelling of soft palate

- Bilateral submandibular swelling (Ludwig's angina)

2. Symptoms of severity

- Severe pain
- Chills
- Difficulty swallowing
- Difficulty breathing
- Malaise

3. Associated problems

- Immunosuppression
- Uncontrolled diabetes
- Prosthetic heart valves
- Reasons for hospital admission are to provide:
- IV antibiotics
- Hydration and rest
- Pain relief
- Extraoral drainage if necessary
- Appropriate monitoring

18 Management of common dental cysts

A cyst may be defined as a radiolucency that is usually fluid-filled and has a lining. The lining is frequently epithelium and in the mouth is either of dental (odontogenic) or non-dental origin (non-odontogenic). A cyst must be differentiated from other pathology that might mimic it, particularly neoplasia.

The common cysts of the jaw arising from epithelium of dental origin are:

1. dental (radicular) or periodontal cysts

2. residual cysts

3. dentigerous cysts

4. eruption cysts

Only the management of the most common cysts in primary care will be discussed here. Please refer to a relevant oral pathology textbook.

Clinical features that may help in differential diagnosis include:

1. History: mode of onset, rate of progression. Cysts are usually slow growing and painless unless secondarily infected. The only cyst that may be painful even if not

infected is the aneurysmal bone cyst which is very rare.

2. Radiographic: consistency and borders - opaque, lucent, mixed, cortication or definition, unilocular or multilocular.

3. Associated teeth: are they vital, non-vital, displaced, resorbed?

4. Bony expansion, resorption, perforation.

5. Location: maxilla, mandible or both. Relation to IDN canal (below or above).

6. Coexistence with other disease (giant cell disease or Gorlin-Goltz syndrome).

Most common cysts seen in a dental practice are radicular cysts or residual cysts (Figures 18.1, 18.2, 18.3). These are usually associated with a non-vital tooth/root or missing tooth. In addition, dentigerous cysts are also common and are associated with impacted teeth (mainly lower wisdom teeth or impacted canines) (Figure 18.4).

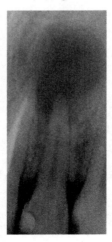

Figure 18.1 Radicular cyst associated with UL2

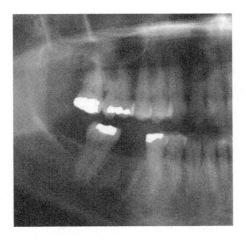

Figure 18.2 Residual cyst LR6

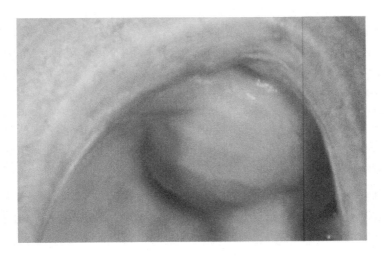

Figure 18.3 Residual cyst in palate of edentulous patient

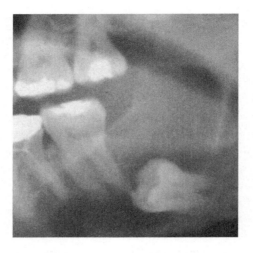

Figure 18.4 Dentigerous cyst associated with impacted LL8

Treatment of a radicular cyst is either by RCT of a non-vital tooth, with or without radicular surgery and enucleation, or extraction of the non-vital tooth and enucleation. It is good practice to send the enucleated lesion off for histopathologic analysis to confirm diagnosis. If the cyst is too large, then it is best to do an incisional biopsy before complete enucleation. If the biopsy confirms odontogenic keratocyst (OKC) then the management is completely different (better refer to hospital).

Aspiration using a large bore needle (eg, white) may aid diagnosis and differentiate between normal anatomy (air), a tumour (empty) or cyst (fluid).

On aspiration, a straw-coloured fluid is pathognomonic of a radicular or residual cyst, whereas aspiration of thick yellow cheesy material is more likely OKC. If you aspirate blood, then this is more likely a vascular malformation of an aneurysmal bone cyst, whereas aspiration of air is an indication of normal anatomy (eg, maxillary sinus).

Cysts are usually asymptomatic unless they become infected or cause displacement of teeth, intra or extraoral swelling, or neurologic symptoms due to pressure on local nerves. Radiographically a radicular cyst appears well defined, unilocular or corticated (depending on duration) unless infected (it then becomes less defined). It is always associated with a non-vital tooth and located above the inferior dental (ID) canal.

What you can do in practice

Take the patient's history (history of old trauma to teeth, decay) and do your usual thorough head and neck examination.

Start with extraoral examination then move on to intraoral, including soft tissue, teeth (colour, decay, vitality, mobility), swelling, expansion or draining sinus, displacement of teeth, missing teeth, root filled teeth, etc.

Take either a radiograph or CBCT (location of lesion and relationship to teeth, roots, impacted or supernumerary teeth, ID canal, relationship to root apex). CBCT for large cysts is more helpful as it reveals the size and relationship to anatomical structures in 3D making the planning of surgical management easier and more predictable.

Aspirate (colour and consistency).

Confirm the diagnosis clinically and radiologically then decide how you are going to treat - with RCT alone or with periradicular surgery. If surgical then do the usual risk assessment.

Risk assessment is paramount and should include asking yourself "Do I have the competence, equipment and the support to deal with the lesion? Is this something that can be done in a primary care setting, or is best referred to hospital due to medical history or the size and nature of the lesion? Do I need to work with the endodontist at the same time, perhaps under IV sedation? Do I have arrangements with a pathology laboratory to analyse the specimen and confirm the diagnosis?".

If the lesion is multilocular, then it is most likely to be OKC or tumour (ameloblastoma) and you should refer to the hospital (Figure 18.5).

Small cysts can usually be curetted or enucleated through the socket after extraction of the root or tooth, whereas for large cysts a flap must be raised to gain adequate access and visibility (Figure 18.6).

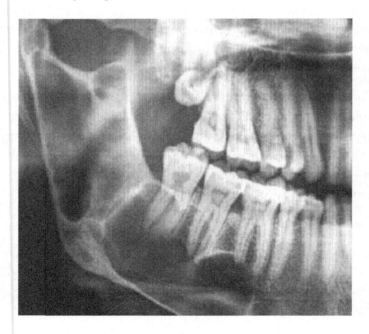

Figure 18.5 Ameloblastoma R mandible

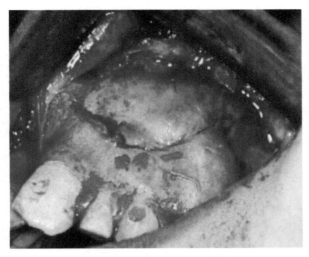

**Figure 18.6 Radicular cyst UL1,2,3
exposed and ready to separate and enucleate**

I usually raise a large three-sided mucoperiosteal flap including at least one tooth either side of the lesion, and carefully remove the bone using a surgical drill and rose head bur. I then separate the cyst from the bony cavity using a large curette or Mitchell's trimmer before I enucleate it and send it off in a formal saline pot to the pathology lab for analysis. I then irrigate with saline and close with 4/0 vicryl rapide sutures. If the cyst is large, I sometimes augment with a suitable synthetic bone graft provided there is no acute infection or pus.

It is better if you work with the endodontist and discuss and manage cases together. Some large cysts can be successfully treated with good endodontic treatment only with the aid of a microscope and a skilled endodontist.

A sensibility test of the involved tooth, and at least one tooth either side of the lesion, should be carried out and documented before any surgical intervention. Always warn the patient that adjacent teeth may lose vitality following enucleation and may require further treatment.

19 Management of common oral lesions in the dental practice

As a clinician, you will come across patients with oral lesions which can be in the form of a lump (sessile or pedunculated), ulcer, fissure, white patch, red lesion or mixed. When you see a lesion in the mouth, it is very important that you go back and ask the patient specifically about the history of the lesion, PMH, any history of trauma or previous surgery, and habits (lip chewing). In addition, some oral lesions can be a manifestation of systemic conditions, for example Crohn's disease, Behcet's syndrome or even HIV.

A. Lesion history

1. How long has the lesion been present? For example, an ulcer that has been there for more than two weeks in a patient with high risk factors should ring alarm bells.

2. Any change in size, shape or colour? A change in colour from white to speckled or red, or a rapid increase in the size of a lump, may indicate malignant transformation.

3. Is the lesion painful?

4. Any altered sensation in the local area? This could be a common symptom of malignancy or a space occupying lesion.

5. Any trauma or oral habits? Lip/cheek biting, smoking, trauma from a sharp tooth or denture? Chemical burn?

6. Any associated features? Fever, malaise, dysphagia?

B. Examination

A thorough extraoral and intraoral examination should be conducted systemically as described in the previous chapter. Describe the lesion in details (site, size, shape, number, colour etc), draw diagrams and take photos. Record positive as well as negative findings. Remember to inspect first then palpate the lesion. If you decide to refer the patient to a specialist or hospital for further management then make sure you include the above findings and attach photos.

Check local lymph glands. Are they raised (as in inflammation or infection)? Number (multiple or solitary)? Tender? Mobile (infection)? Fixed (malignancy)?

C. Clinical judgement

Think before you cut. Once all the information has been collected and a differential diagnosis has been made, a management strategy should be formulated and executed. For example, if you suspect an ulcer is caused by trauma from a sharp tooth or denture, then smoothing or filling of the sharp fragment and a waiting period of no longer than two weeks should be implemented. If it was trauma-induced, then it should heal within this time period. If however the lesion does not heal, then a biopsy or urgent hospital referral may be considered to confirm the diagnosis and exclude malignancy.

If the lesion is small, painless, has been present for many years with no increase in size and is not bothering the patient, then take photos and monitor.

20 Oral biopsy

This is the removal of tissue, cells or fluid from a living body for diagnostic examination in order to establish or confirm diagnosis of disease. It is important that general dentists working in primary care realise their important role in cancer detection and management. Any dentist should be able to perform a biopsy for clinically benign-looking lesions (eg, lichen planus, Figure 20.1).

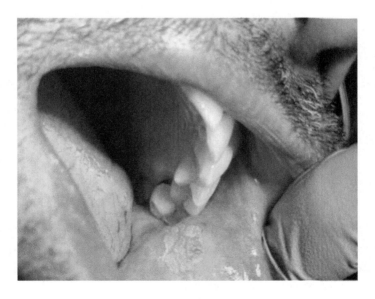

Figure 20.1 Lichen planus L cheek

You should have an arrangement with a local hospital either privately or through the NHS. However, a biopsy should not be performed in a primary care setting for lesions highly suspicious of oral cancer. Instead, the patient should be urgently referred to the local hospital for investigation and management. It is easier for the specialist to evaluate and examine the tissue in an undisturbed state rather than a touched and/or incised state. Furthermore, incision of the lesion in a primary care setting may stimulate proliferation and spread and worsen the prognosis (Figure 20.2).

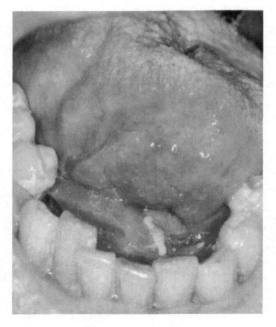

Figure 20.2 SCC floor of mouth

It is better if you urgently call your local maxillofacial or oral medicine department and formally refer the patient including the result of your history and examination and any photos or radiographs.

Most common types of biopsies are incisional, excisional,

punch and aspiration. Size, character and radiographic finding determines the type of biopsy.

A. Incisional biopsy

It is the gold standard for large lesions and is used to establish a definitive diagnosis before initiating final treatment. Here a small piece of abnormal tissue is removed, ideally including a small part of clinically normal tissue. The biopsy should be deep and narrow rather than wide and shallow. This is to ensure all thickness of the mucosa is included and the deeper layers are not missed (usually the superficial layer is necrotic and non-diagnostic, and the deeper layers are usually where the cancer cellular changes are).

Usually, infiltration anaesthesia around the area is sufficient. Using a 15c blade take a wedge (two elliptical incisions, Figure 20.3) from the area which shows most clinical change, and send the specimen in a pot (Figure 20.4) containing 10% formal saline to the pathology laboratory. Include the patient's details, site of specimen, clinical information, and suspected diagnosis (Figure 20.5).

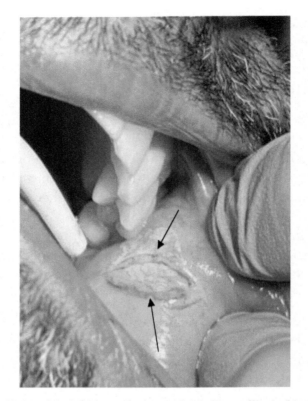

Figure 20.3 Incisional biopsy lesion L cheek (Two elliptical incisions including a small area of normal tissue)

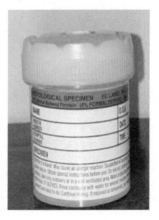

Figure 20.4 showing biopsy pot containing 10% formal saline

Figure 20.5 showing a sample of the pathology form
which is sent to the lab with the biopsy pot

B. Excisional biopsy

The whole lesion is excised fully, including 1-2mm of the clinically normal tissue below and around the lesion, and sent to the lab. This is usually indicated for small clinically-looking benign lesions with no sinister features (eg, polyp, or mucocele, Figures 20.6 and 20.7).

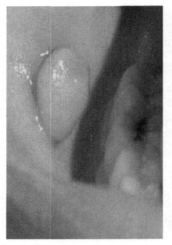
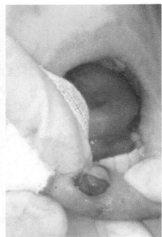

Figure 20.6   Figure 20.7

Fibroepithelial polyp R cheek   Mucocele lower lip

It is also used for obviously clinically benign lesions that are large (eg, odontogenic cyst, Figure 20.8).

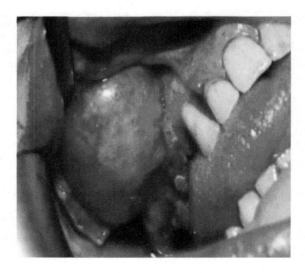

Figure 20.8 Enucleation of a radicular cyst UR4,5,6

C. Aspiration biopsy

This is the removal of some contents of the lesion for quick observation. It is usually performed chair side using a large pore needle (18 gauge) and a 5 to 10cc syringe. It is useful in ruling out if the lesion is vascular or otherwise. If you aspirate air then maybe the lesion is a sinus or traumatic bone cyst, or if yellow (pus), the straw-coloured fluid may indicate a dental cyst. Thick cheesy material may indicate an odontogenic keratocyst (OKC), and if there is no aspirate then the lesion may be solid (tumour). If you aspirate blood, then keep away.

This is different to FNAC (analysing cells) where aspirate is sent to the lab for cytological analysis, which will not be discussed here.

D. Punch biopsy

I only included this for completion, but I do not prefer it. I think if a biopsy is warranted then it is better to take a proper one rather than crush the tissue and obtain a small, possibly non-diagnostic specimen.

21 Quiz

Q1. A 70-year-old retired man presents to your dental surgery as an emergency complaining of severe dental pain from his lower right jaw (pain score 9-10). It has been there for a few days and is severe, throbbing and is not relieved by NSAID. The pain is aggravated by hot drinks.

PMH includes type 1 diabetes, osteoporosis and atrial fibrillation (AF). His medications include insulin, metformin, warfarin and he has just started taking alendronic acid tablets. He is a non-smoker and is not allergic to any known medications. He gave a history of failed local anaesthesia at his dentist a few years ago and is therefore nervous.

O/E: he has right sided mild facial swelling, slight erythema and his mouth opening is slightly reduced. He has free tongue movement, and his floor of mouth is soft. His right submandibular lymph nodes are slightly enlarged and tender. His temperature is slightly high at 37.8 degrees, and he feels unwell.

His lower right second premolar and first molar are unrestorable, grade 1 mobile and very TTP (Figure 21.1).

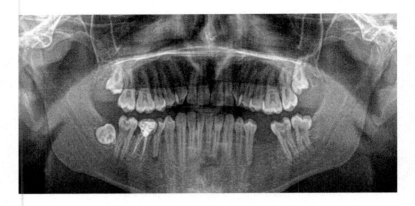

Figure 21.1 LR5,6 unrestorable

He also has a lacy white, reticular patch in his R cheek, which is smooth, 2x2 cm in diameter adjacent to heavily amalgam restored UR6 (Figure 21.2). He was unaware of this lesion, however, he mentioned that he also has skin rashes and a white patch on his genital area.

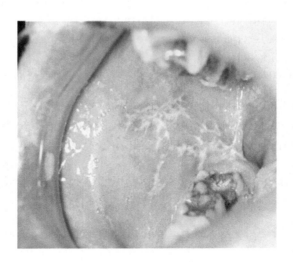

Figure 21.2 White patch R cheek

A. What is your diagnosis?

B. How would you manage this case?

Q2. You qualified as a dentist last year, and you have extracted a very limited number of teeth as most of what you do daily in your dental practice is general and cosmetic dentistry. You have already spent 30 minutes extracting a very difficult carious and heavily restored UR7 for a healthy 60-year-old man under LA and the tooth snapped. Half of the palatal root broke off. The tooth was carious and painful but there was no acute infection or abscess. The patient became anxious and nervous. There was no plan to replace the tooth with an implant as it is a back tooth, and the patient can't afford implants. The radiograph that you already have reveals a very close proximity to the sinus.

A. How would you manage this case?

Q3. You have successfully extracted a carious tooth for an 80-year-old lady. However, she came back to your surgery a few hours later with profuse bleeding from the extraction socket. She was accompanied by her daughter who reported that her mum had lost a fair amount of blood, and she feels weak and tired. She also mentioned that her mum takes blood thinners, but she can't remember the name.

A. What do you think is the cause of her bleeding?

B. How would you manage this case?

Please email your answer to abdul@yorkshiredentalsuite.co.uk.

That's it then – at least for this book! As I said in my introduction, my aim in writing it is to pass on tips from the knowledge gained during my vast experience in oral surgery. It is aimed at junior dentists and dentists with a special interest in oral surgery. I hope you have learned something from reading it, and that I have given you the confidence to try out some of my techniques. I wish you every success as your dental career continues.

Good luck!

Dr Abdul Dalghous

Acknowledgements

First and foremost, I would like to thank God for giving me wisdom, guidance and knowledge. Also, my wife Dr Afaf El-Hamidi, my twin sons Dr Hassan and Dr Hussein, my son Mohammed and my youngest son Ali, for their patience and support during the writing of this book. In addition, Dr Mark Spencer, a friend and mentor, for his valuable advice and support; Carole Kendal for her help with proofreading this book; the amazing team at Yorkshire Dental Suite; and Rosy, for the diagrammatic artwork and illustrations.

Printed in Great Britain
by Amazon

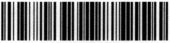